MW01156540

WHEN HE WAS ANNA

A MOM'S JOURNEY INTO THE TRANSGENDER
WORLD

PATTI HORNSTRA

KWE
PUBLISHING, LLC

Hornstra, Patti. *When He Was Anna: A Mom's Journey Into the Transgender World.*

Copyright © 2020 by Patti Hornstra

Published by KWE Publishing: www.kwepub.com

All rights reserved.

ISBNs 978-1-950306-38-1 (paperback) and 978-1-950306-39.8 (ebook).

Library of Congress Control Number: 2020907797

Cover photo by Todd Trapani, Trapaniphotography.com

Cover photo modifications by Mallory Hornstra, malloryhornstradesign.com

This book is dedicated to Tristan.
I'm so glad that God sent you. You filled the empty chair at the table.

FOREWORD

Raising children is work. They are work from the time they are born until the time their parents leave the earth. It's ironic that we refer to them as a "bundle of joy" when they are born. There is certainly joy during the parenting journey, but that joy is mixed with so many other emotions as well. Our parents felt the same mix of emotions when they were raising us, but some of the issues our parents dealt with when we were growing up are so different than what parents deal with today. I think it started with Adam and Eve, and it has not stopped since.

It seems that society is becoming more complex—and more problematic. There are so many new social norms that are begging to be accepted. We have new terms, like "politically correct" or "PC," to add to our new vocabulary. Society encourages us to be "PC" in order to keep everyone on the same track. Being "PC" means reining in those people who may struggle to accept the new ways of thinking and speaking. Being "PC" means that we may have to adjust what we do/say/believe in order to fit in with today's society. But, it's not all bad. Some of these new norms are good and some are not.

Parents today face many more challenges than ever before.

When I was four years old, kids were making mud pies. Today a four-year-old is putting apps on their parents' phones. In elementary school, we worried about cooties. Today we worry about everything from peanut allergies to autism, and the list goes on. The world has changed.

When Patti told me that she wanted to write a book about Tristan and tell her story about this journey into the transgender world, I was honestly surprised. Patti is a very private person. She fixes problems (she was a handler long before Showtime's *Ray Donovan* came along). Like most mothers, she will go to battle for her kids and wants to help them navigate this world in a way that most mothers will understand. You don't poke the mama bear. Mothers are the ones who bring children into the world. Yes, dad might be the Lamaze coach, but that's nothing like giving birth—sorry, dudes.

This book is about a mother's journey when her sixteen-year-old daughter, the youngest of four, announced that she was transgender. This book does not celebrate that fact, nor does it condemn it. This book is about the love a parent has for their child. It's about a parent who wants to support their child but who also struggles in a rapidly changing world. This book is about the frustration of trying to navigate a system of medical doctors and therapists who take the path of least resistance rather than step back and dig deeper to really diagnose the issue. There are many good medical professionals and therapists out there but, just like every other profession, there are some who do more harm than good.

Patti wanted to write this book to let other parents know that they are not alone in their frustration as they struggle to accept what society tells us is now normal. It's okay to feel the hurt and anger that comes along with that frustration. It's okay to have questions. It's okay not to be politically correct in today's society.

This story is about a parent's love for a child.

Patti does a remarkable job of explaining this journey using raw, unapologetic emotions. This story is real, warts and all. I know because I was there the whole time. I'm Tristan's dad, the other part of Team Eleven (that will make sense later). I know we are not the only ones out there who are living this story, the only message in a bottle wondering if anyone else is out there.

Patti asked me if I wanted to read the book as she was writing it, and I declined. She does a much better job of writing than I ever could, and I didn't want to interject something that would influence her explanation of how she felt, how we felt. I'm just the Lamaze coach.

Peace to all as you go through your own journey,

Curtis Hornstra

AUTHOR'S NOTE

Personally, I NEVER read the preface or the introduction to a book. Reading about the author's *inspiration*, their *motivation*, *blah blah blah*, always seemed just a little too touchy-feely for me. But it's funny what you figure out when you decide to dump your feelings onto a page in hopes that someone else will read about them (thank you for that). You learn that what comes before the story is likely *part* of the story, and you should *read* it if you want to *get* it. So please read it.

PREFACE

Hi, I'm Patti H., and I'm the mother of a transgender child.

Other than that, my life is now, and has always been, wonderful yet largely unremarkable. I've been married to the most amazing man since 1987, and we have four equally amazing children. God has blessed me with a wonderful life filled with love. If the God reference isn't "PC" and offends you, I'm sorry—but not really. If you read beyond this paragraph, then you'll see that my story is anything but politically correct.

You're sure to see God come up again, and you'll hopefully read things that make you say, "I can't believe she said that." That's the point here—raw truth, no bullshit. I'm going to tell it like it is, from my perspective, like it or not, agree with it or not—it's the truth. You can applaud me, you can call me nasty names, and whatever emotion creeps up as you read my story is okay with me. My feelings are mine without apology.

I am not a therapist nor am I a specialist on anything to do with gender (gender dysphoria, gender fluidity, or transgenderness, if that's even a word). This is not a self-help book, nor is it intended to be. Lord knows, I have a hard-enough time helping myself. What

I'm writing is simply a chronology, a timeline of my journey as the mom of a transgender child (yes, teen, but she/he will ALWAYS be my child). I don't even know what to call myself, not that I'm looking for a label. But, let's face it, I'm not a transgender mom. That seems to connote that I'm a mom who's transgender. So, I'm just a mom of a transgender child. But, I'm the mom of three non-transgender children, too. I love each of my kids as much as the others. I love them for their uniqueness, for their kindness, and for their talents. I could burst with pride at what great people all *four* have grown to be, despite the seven million mistakes I made along the way. But, Christopher, Mallory, and Andrew—none of you have presented me with a life situation where I needed to write a book to work through it. That distinction belongs to Number Four, the one I named Anna Marie who now goes by Tristan Blaine. I don't think that events or situations in your life define you (so there you go, I don't even need a label), but they certainly help to shape you.

First things first, then. Please go back and read the line above the last paragraph, the part that says, "I'm the mom of a transgender *child.*" I say "child," because frankly, deep down inside, I still don't get it. The emotional struggle remains. Do I have a transgender daughter or a transgender son? My child was born a girl and announced at age sixteen that she was a boy (much more to come in the following chapters). So, which is it—transgender daughter or transgender son? I know there's a right and wrong here, but that part still confuses the hell out of me, even after two years. (For the record, according to the terminology, I technically have a transgender son, a female at birth who identifies as a male.)

So here it is, my selfish rant about the trauma of trying to parent a transgender child, or really a transgender teenager. *Trying* is the operative word here. As you'll soon find out, I have no idea what I'm doing. Mistakes? Oh honey, I've made more than my share. I'm a mess on so many transgender parenting levels. And so I've decided to give myself a pass, just for this one time. I'm going to unapologetically spill it all. Remember, this whole thing is about my feelings, my struggles, my heartache. No bullshit. If you've been through something similar you might think, "Finally, someone said what I've wanted to say." Or maybe you'll just think I'm a cold-hearted nut, or a total loser, or just an awful mom. Whatever you think is just fine with me. Your feelings and opinions are yours without apology, too.

ACKNOWLEDGMENTS

There is no greater agony than bearing an untold story inside you.

~ Maya Angelou

In the early days of our journey, Tristan suggested that I find a therapist to help me work through the confusion and complicated mix of emotions that had suddenly become my world. While I appreciated the suggestion, traditional therapy just wasn't my thing. I was certain that I could work through all of this on my own. After two years divine intervention pointed me in the right direction. God let me know that I needed to write this book—it was my therapy. My lifelong dream of writing a book finally came through, but certainly not in a way I had ever imagined. Sharing my personal struggles and failures was never part of the plan, but here I am doing just that. I'm so thankful that He knew what I needed when I didn't. And I'm especially thankful for the people He's chosen to bring into my life.

Thank you . . .

Curtis Lee—you're the love of my life, my number one

Christopher, Mallory, Andrew, and Tristan—you've grown into extraordinary adults, and I could not be more proud of each of you

Tristan's Grandparents: Darrell, Maxine, Michael—you've shown nothing but grace and acceptance throughout this journey of ours

Those Very Few Friends With Whom I've Shared This—your support has meant more to me than you could possibly know

Kim, KWE Publishing—your guidance has been invaluable

INTRODUCTION

My mom used to tell a story about going to see a palm reader (I am not joking) when I was a toddler. Madame Sophia—I'm calling her that because I have no idea what her name was, and because that sounds like a cool name for a palm reader—told my mom a lot of stuff, some about her and some about me. The part about me: I'd marry a man whose name began with an "H," I'd have a long, happy marriage, she thought I'd have three kids (she said that part was fuzzy for her), and I would write books. That was about fifty years ago (I feel so old), and it looks like Madame S. was pretty much spot on.

The three kids thing was unclear for her, but it was pretty unclear for me, too. My husband was one of four kids (two boys, two girls, all in less than five years). I was an only child. Like a classic only child, I wanted the opposite of what I had. I wanted a BIG family. To an only, four kids is definitely big. So, I wanted four. The first two came pretty easily; we decided to have a baby, and nine months later, voilà! We were on a roll, and I wanted number three right on the heels of number two. But number three took a little longer—a shocking two and a half years for Andrew to get here. By that time, I was twenty-nine and tired—three kids in four and a half years is no small adventure. Do the mom math: two hands + three little kids = a lot to handle. So, Curt and I decided that three would have to be it. And so, we were a family of five. A family of five at a six-top kitchen table. And that was the problem for me. I looked at that empty chair and wondered who was supposed to be sitting in it.

CHAPTER 1

THE NUMBERS

I am your Creator. You were in my care even before you were born.

~ Isaiah 44:2a (CEV)

December 1999 was a great end to a great year. Andrew (number three, my Christmas-time baby) turned five, which meant all day preschool. Kindergarten was looming on the horizon; diaper bags and car seats were long gone. In 1999 you didn't have to keep kids in car seats until they started middle school, which I'm pretty sure is the law in at least forty-eight states as of now. I was thirty-four, Curt was thirty-nine, life was good! We lived in an upscale suburban neighborhood in a big house with some awesome neighbors. Y2K was on everyone's mind, so we decided it was time to *party like it's 1999* (if you don't get that reference then I have no words).

How does a neighborhood of thirty somethings party like it's 1999? You have parties. December 18 was a fancy progressive dinner, and it was a blast; by the dessert course, we had people falling out of their chairs. I was among those who kept their seat. And the grand finale? On New Year's Eve 1999, we joined two hundred of our closest friends (black tie, private invitation only) in my neighbor's backyard two doors down from our house. We tented their backyard, hired a DJ, a caterer, waitstaff, a bartender, you get the picture.

On to January 2000. I felt crappy, achy, couldn't sleep, just yuck. For weeks. My boobs hurt, my back hurt, and even after already having three kids it never occurred to me that I might be pregnant. Birth control pills always work, right? (Side note: We're Catholic, and that's relevant since here come the church references. Don't worry, I'm religious but not a religious fanatic, and this isn't an attempt to convert you or to convince you that I'm a perfect Catholic—which I'm not. Look, I just admitted that I took birth control pills.)

On Saturday, January 29 (Y2K), we went to 5:30 pm Mass. Being Catholic is awesome because you can go to church on Saturday night if there's something big you needed to deal with on Sunday like a "Big Football Game" or a snowstorm, both of which were coming up the next day. I saw my doctor at Mass, and since she was a dear friend as well as a church buddy, we went into the ladies' room to try and figure out why I felt so awful. She suggested a pregnancy test (wait until Sunday morning for best results, she said), and I thought she'd lost her mind. Remember, I'd already had three kids—what kind of idiot has three kids and doesn't know she's pregnant again? That would be me. Since I wasn't sleeping (at all, for weeks) I decided that 2:00 am was a good time to take that pregnancy test. You've figured out the rest. Since it was 2:00 am and I couldn't call my doctor/friend, I decided to wake up Curt and share the shock. And that's what it was, shock. Not bad, just shock. You see, I'd had a private talk with God, ongoing for months, and had told him that I still saw that empty chair at the table, and I wondered if it wasn't time to fill that seat. I had no idea He was going to answer.

Back to the "Big Football Game"/snowstorm. "Big Football Game #34" (I can't put the real name in the book without paying royalties) started at 6:25 pm Eastern Time, and the snow had been coming down for hours. I couldn't have cared less, because I was sixteen hours into my "what in the hell just happened" zone. The Tennessee Titans played the Los Angeles Rams, the latter of which happened to be my husband's favorite team. So here we are, all 5.2 of us, ready to watch Dad's favorite team. And then the power went out. And then the panic set in. My panic. I really have no idea where Curt was emotionally at this point, all I remember is that he REALLY wanted to see that football game. As much as he loves jumping in the car, risking life and limb in a snowstorm *just because he can*, Curt knew that he'd better stay put. No sports bar "Big Football Game" for him. He got out the sleeping bags, turned on the gas fireplace, and camped out in the family room with three kids. While they camped, all snug as bugs, I worked on night number forty-two of sleeplessness, which sadly has grown to a total of 7,296 sleepless nights as of this writing. I have my own math system, you know, and if you take nine months of pregnancy without sleep, add 19.25 years of parenting this child without sleep, then the sum is 7,296 sleepless nights. The silver lining in all this sleeplessness was that it gave me more time to panic! I could now panic all day AND all night.

That night, I was in full panic mode about one thing only—Andrew would NEVER get to Disney World. We'd taken Christopher and Mallory to Disney World a few years back, but Andrew stayed behind since he was barely one and a half (he stayed with Grandma and Grandpa, in case you were wondering). My plan had been to take him to Disney when he was five or six, which gave me over a year to plan it and get it done. All I could think of that night was that I was pregnant, Andrew had just turned five, Christopher and Mallory had already been to Disney World, and now Andrew would never, ever in his whole life see Mickey. I then did the most rational thing I could think of. I got a paper, pen, and a flashlight (no power, and it was dark) and called the Disney reservation number. I could not have found a more expensive way to book that trip if I'd tried, but we went to Disney World for Mother's Day 2000.

Snow melts, the "Big Football Game" ends (the Rams won), February rolls in, and life goes back to normal. Sort of. Time to figure out the details. I assumed I was a couple of weeks pregnant by the first of February. We're in mid-February now, and I'm thinking this will be an October baby. Two OB-GYN visits and one ultrasound later, my doctor says the funniest thing to me: "It looks like your EDC (that's what the doc called your due date back in the olden days, your *estimated date of confinement*) is September 10." He then pauses to look at the conception calendar/wheel. "That would make your date of conception December 18. Anything memorable about that day?" I laughed until I almost peed my pants. Don't get it? Go back a few paragraphs and you will.

My October baby was really a September baby; I was about eight weeks pregnant before I even had a clue.

TABLE FOR SIX

Having four kids grants you instant access to the exclusive club known as "Wow, That's a Lot of Kids!" I couldn't wait. I already had more kids than I had hands, so what was one more? The empty seat at the table would be filled, and all would be right with the world. This baby may have been a surprise, but boy was she wanted—and celebrated! This child, number four, was everybody's baby. My neighbor buddies (most with babies neither in the house nor on the horizon) couldn't wait for our little bundle of joy to arrive. My other three kids were thrilled, particularly Andrew who saw the new baby as the end to his days as the youngest child in the family (plus this was his ticket to Disney World). And Curt? Well, he had told me (many times) after Andrew was born that if we ever had another child, we were selling the big suburban house and moving to a farm. He grew up as one of four, and he apparently thought that only farmers and crazy people had more than three kids. As fate would have it, the suburbs won out and I was able to stay in suburbia. Curt never bought us that farm, but he did buy me a fancy new mini-van two days after Anna was born. He needed to make sure his princess (the baby, not me) had safe transportation.

CHAPTER 2

THE BAND

Everything in high school seems like the most important thing
that's ever happened in your life. It's not.
You'll get out of high school and you never see those people again.
All the people who torment and press you
won't make a difference in your life in the long haul.

~ Mark Hoppus, Blink-182

You likely can't tell yet, but this mama's a planner (i.e., control freak). I'm scheduled, organized, on track—except for pregnancy number four. I had missed twenty percent of prime planning time; forty pregnancy weeks, eight weeks without a clue. The next seven months were a whirlwind of planning for this baby who was surprising me and keeping me on my toes since before we even knew she was coming. She had a name as soon as we knew her gender (back then there were two genders, and control freak moms needed to know which one was on the way). The name I chose was Tessa (it means fourth child, if you want to look it up), but Curt was having none of that, so she was crowned Anna Marie. And she was the cutest little brown-haired, brown-eyed princess you've ever seen! And she was exhausting. From the moment she was born she seemed to be on a mission to control everyone and everything in her range. She was the *mistress of all she surveyed* (if that line is familiar then you were born before 1970 and you heard it from Susan Lucci on *All My Children*, forever one of my favorite television quotes).

Anna Marie was personable, outgoing, smart as a whip—really a leader in any/every situation in which she found herself. She's the only (and I do mean only) child I know whose pre-kindergarten teacher insisted that she NOT be held back a year and instead start kindergarten a few days before her fifth birthday. Back in the old days (1990s and 2000s) they (the parents, the pre-k teachers, the kindergarten teachers) always wanted you to hold the kids in pre-K until they were six years old or close to it. And here we were sending our baby off to the cold hard world of kindergarten and she wasn't even going to turn five for a few days; I'm still surprised that Child Protective Services didn't pay us a visit. I often wonder— secretly until now—if I made a mistake by not holding her back a year. I wonder if it would have made a difference when she got older, if the happy, outgoing Anna Marie from kindergarten would have still turned into the depressed, introverted Anna Marie who appeared in middle school. Hindsight, but who knows.

So, middle school. Three lost years of trying to fit in, make friends, keep friends, wear the right clothes, say the right things, not eat lunch alone, wonder why no one likes you, wonder why adults are such idiots, wonder why you're the only one struggling with all of it. Parental hell. I had been in parental hell before, three times, but this was the hell of a different making. This hell changed my child. She had band to keep her busy (trumpet was her instrument of choice in middle school, more about that later), and she had friends. But she wasn't the leader of the pack anymore. She left that behind and became the follower to end all followers. My Bon Jovi-loving cutie (we had even surprised her at Christmas when she was nine years old with tickets to see JBJ in Washington DC) went dark. Dark clothes, dark eye liner, dark music. You like screaming, indecipherable, head banging music? You wear all dark, head to toe, military boots and all? If that's all it took to be your friend, then she was in! I hated it, but I knew how to play the game: keep a close eye on the friends, try not to sweat the clothes, know that parents usually hate their kids' music . . . you get it. I looked for the light at the end of the tunnel. I was certain that it was only a phase, that she'd grow out of it. And I waited. Sixth grade. Seventh grade. Eighth grade. Somehow, I thought that high school would be the magic bullet to leave the darkness of middle school behind. Onward and upward, bigger and better things, I was waiting for the cliché gods to swoop in and save the day.

There was no swooping, there was no saving, and high school brought with it more of the same. At first, I thought there might be a reprieve from the dark days of middle school since Anna's love of music continued, and she joined the marching band. Band meant new friends, uniforms, and Dinkles (marching band shoes) instead of combat boots. You can see why I was hopeful! Band kids aren't known for their dark side, so brighter days were on the horizon! She went from trumpet to mellophone (a marching French horn in case you didn't know), and band was now her life's true passion. (Important side note here: if I had to choose one word to describe Anna it would be passionate. If I had to choose more words they would be dedicated, intense, focused, brilliant—yes, I know that 99.9% of the parents in my upper-middle-class bubble think their kids are brilliant, but this one really is.)

Marching band turned out to be both a blessing and a curse. If you don't know much about marching band, then let me fill you in. It's a lifestyle, not only for the band kids, but for their families as well. She became a band kid; I became a band mom. Home life revolved around the band schedule. These kids are together every weekday, and they often travel together for competitions (with parental chaperones, can you say Disney World?!?!) outside of school hours. What happens when marching season is over? Well, then there's concert band! For the most part, the same kids in marching band are in concert band—plus, the girls get to wear a black dress and black shoes to perform in concert band. Score for Anna!

Anna did make band friends, but she was pretty demanding of them. Band was her baby, and she took it quite seriously. The other fifty-plus kids in the marching band—not always so much. Some shared a similar passion; others saw band as just another elective. It was frustrating for her to spend so much time with kids who were less passionate that she was. She was quite vocal about their flippant disregard for all things marching band, which often led to alienation—hers from them. Her guidance counselor summed it up perfectly for Anna during one of their counseling sessions to discuss her frustration with the lack of seriousness among her band peers. She told Anna that band was her (Anna's) baby, and that she got to choose how to parent her baby. But for the other band kids, band is their baby, too, and they get to choose how to parent their baby. I thought this analogy was quite wise, and I was sorry I didn't think of it; the single, twenty-five-year-old guidance counselor out-parented me on that one.

And so, band was her absolute life's passion—until it wasn't. In her three years of high school she ate, slept, and breathed band. (Let's stop here and see if you're paying attention. THREE years of high school. She started high school in the ninth grade—what happened to the fourth year? Well, you've read this far so you'll need to keep going to read about that twist and turn.) She marched with a mellophone, played French horn in concert band, dabbled in trumpet and drums—with the appropriate lessons for each of these along the way. Did I say yet that everything revolved around band? How do you stay close to your high school-aged band kid? You become a band mom. You chaperone trips; make friends with the other band moms; set up props at football games, then run them onto the field for performances; and sell pizza and chicken sandwiches at the concession stand, end up in charge of the concession stand, and bring your kid vegetarian chicken patties for dinner before every game (because she's a vegetarian and you want her to have something to eat since the only choice for the band kids is Chick-fil-A). I'm serious about that. Ask any band kid in the free world what the band moms bring in for them to eat before the performances and you'll get the same answer: Chick-fil-A.

Now, what's a band kid to do when it's time to up the game? When the high school band leaves you longing for more? *You apply to march with a competitive marching corps!!* Let me explain. During tenth grade, my still fourteen-year-old announced that she wanted to apply to march with a competitive drum corps. This is like marching band on steroids. In true Anna fashion, she was a dog with a bone, and her obsession du jour was marching drum corps. Marching band kids from all over the world apply to march with a corps of their choosing, and if accepted they spend about eleven weeks of the summer traveling around the country and performing. The crowning glory is DCI's (Drum Corps International) competition in August at Lucas Oil Stadium in Indianapolis. It's the "Big Game" of marching band where the top twenty-five corps come together and compete for three days. It also meant that Anna, if accepted, would be gone for eleven weeks, traveling to over a dozen states, and sleeping in gymnasiums with two hundred other band kids in her corps. I was terrified, so of course I said no way. But, in true Anna fashion (the child with an uncanny knack for convincing you to do things that you swear you'll never do), she found a way to make it happen. That summer, after tenth grade, the two of us took a trip to witness DCI firsthand. I wanted/needed to see up close and personal what this thing was all about. It was a great trip. After checking it out for a few days and badgering dozens of other band moms from all over the U.S., I was satisfied that Anna would be in good hands if she earned a spot in next year's corps. I was also satisfied that the likelihood of her earning a spot for the next year (she would be barely sixteen years old when she auditioned the next fall) was practically nil; everyone assured me that marching corps rarely accept sixteen-years-olds. Win/win for Mom.

Eleventh grade started off with a bang. School started almost as soon as we got home from DCI. Anna was nervous, excited, and worked her butt off. She was going to audition in October for a spot with the Colts, a corps in Iowa, so she was in full-on prep mode which included private mellophone lessons to get her in top shape for her audition. In October the two of us flew to Dubuque, Iowa; I checked in at the Holiday Inn and she checked in to the floor of the gym with a new blowup mattress and a bundle of nerves. (Side note: who in the hell wants to leave Virginia and go to Iowa in October? October in Virginia is practically still summer; October in Iowa found me at JCPenney buying fuzzy warm socks.) It was a proud mama moment. My introverted, *get-away-from-me-but-don't-leave-my-side,* barely sixteen-year-old jumped in and took control of her destiny. She wanted it, and she was going after it. I was simply scared and confused by the whole thing. Secretly, I was relieved that she had two strikes against her from what "they" all said: she was barely sixteen and this was her first audition, so she had virtually no chance of being offered a contract. Looking back, I think she must have known all along that she was going to make this happen. She even met with her high school principal before the audition to discuss her options since she'd be missing one Friday each month to fly to Iowa and would miss the last three weeks of school if she got a contract. He was great, and told her to go for it with the full support of the school should she get a spot with the corps. Let's just jump to the end of the weekend, where—you guessed it—she was offered a contract.

And so began the family fun of flying to Iowa one weekend every month from October through January (the two of us; Curt joined us in January since she insisted that he experience a corps weekend in person). We'd leave on Friday morning, land in Dubuque Friday in the late afternoon, pick up the rental car, drive to the hotel to drop off my bags (with the obligatory snow storms thrown in a couple of times), drive her to the gymnasium of the weekend (they varied depending on what middle school/high school/concert venue was available at the time), and drop her off. Then I'd spend the rest of the weekend either working from the hotel room (computers really are amazing, aren't they) or playing parent-volunteer with the corps. On Sunday afternoon I'd pick her up from corps, head to the airport, and fly home until we did it again in four weeks. Starting in February she began to fly alone. I was convinced after four trips together that she could handle the Chicago layover like a pro (she could find an airport Starbucks like a homing pigeon, so what else was left in successful airport navigation?), and I wanted her to get used to the independence that she'd have all summer when she marched with the Colts. The process operated like a well-oiled machine. By this point I'd witnessed the Colts staff picking up members at the airport a bunch of times, and I knew that she'd be in good hands when she landed in Iowa. So, I'd see her off on Friday, spend the weekend like a Nervous Nellie, then pick her up on Sunday evening to hear about the adventures of the weekend. Needless to say, the months flew by. They were a whirlwind of band practice, performances, private lessons, and trips to Iowa.

May of Anna's junior year arrived way too quickly. Suddenly this thing was real. Amazon boxes were a daily fixture on the front porch. A summer with drum corps means traveling light, but it's amazing how much stuff you need to buy to travel light. I'm still trying to figure that one out. You get to take one suitcase, a very specific size. You need these shorts in this particular color (and you need at least eight pair because you do laundry every two weeks—if you're lucky), so many socks, toiletries for the entire summer, you get the picture—all packed up tight in the special-sized suitcase. Then there's the air mattress that doesn't cut it once it arrives and the lightweight travel cot to replace the disappointing air mattress, then the other lightweight travel cot to replace the first lightweight travel cot that also didn't quite cut it. Oh, and the very specific brand and style of shoes for practice—two pair, and you sure can't get those at Costco. Let's just say that, between lightweight travel cots and special (read: expensive) shoes, we got to know REI almost as well as we got to know the Amazon driver.

Anna was nervous, excited, grumpy, and ecstatic, all at the same time. She finished her last three weeks of classwork early (public school in much of Virginia typically goes through mid-June), put junior year behind her, and flew to Dubuque on the Friday before Memorial Day. She'd be gone for eleven weeks. We made plans to see her perform a few times (two performances in Pennsylvania and Virginia were doable, and Florida was a possibility). Curt and I would drive a rental car one way to Indianapolis in August for DCI, then the three of us would fly back to Virginia together. We knew that the eleven weeks would fly by, and we were all (nervously) excited for her adventure. The plan was perfection, until it wasn't.

THE BLACK BELT

Anna had always marched to her own beat (pun intended), and her beat was intense. She loved what she loved with all of the passion and obsession that she could muster, and she hated what she hated with even more of the same. Even as a tiny little girl, she had a mind of her own and was stubborn as a mule. She liked going with me when I took the other three kids to whatever activity they were involved in. That was a good thing for both of us since, as a little kid with three older siblings, she had no choice but to tag along and make the best of it. We strapped her in her car seat, drove to the activity du jour, and she played where she was planted. By the time she was four she spent a lot of time planted (with me) in the lobby of the karate studio where Andrew, then about ten years old, had started taking martial arts classes. Anna had a blast playing in the waiting room, but the instructor (a big beefy sweetheart of a guy who thought she was adorable and always said "hi" to her) with his black *gi* (karate uniform) and black belt seemed to intimidate the daylights out of her. This went on several times each week for a few years. And then one day he didn't intimidate the daylights out of her anymore. She decided that she liked him, and she liked karate, and playing dolls in the waiting room wasn't going to cut it for her anymore. In fact, she decided that if Andrew could get his Black Belt (which he had) then she could get hers (which she did).

CHAPTER 3
THE COLTS

Life is about choices. Some we regret, some we're proud of. Some will haunt us forever. The message - we are what we chose to be.

~ Graham Brown

The *I Can Fly to Iowa Alone* plan included a phone call home as soon as the plane landed; Anna was really good about this. She's a rule follower, after all, and she called every month as soon as she landed. The May phone call came in like clockwork, but this time it was different. As soon as Anna called, she asked if Curt and I would fly to Iowa for the weekend. This was her eighth trip there, and her fourth trip alone, so it was odd since she'd handled every other Iowa weekend like a champ. She sounded okay, assured us that nothing was wrong, and that she just wanted us to come for the weekend. The answer was no. There was no way that Curt and I were hopping on a plane to Dubuque at the last minute over Memorial Day weekend, knowing full well that as soon as we got there she'd be off with her buds and we'd be left watching the

Oxygen Channel at the local Holiday Inn. And so, we stayed in Virginia. I'd love to just end it here and say that she got over her angst super quickly and we all had a wonderful summer with an amazing reunion in August at DCI. And I'd love to say that I didn't spend the weekend hiding my tears and wishing I were at the Holiday Inn in Dubuque, Iowa watching the Oxygen Channel. But I promised honesty, so here it is in all its (sometimes childish) ugliness.

The airport call was the first of a string of calls over the next three days. Calls from Anna. Calls from the corps director, Deidre. Lots and lots of calls. So many calls in three days. She wanted to come home, she didn't want to come home. Nothing was wrong. She just missed home. Then she wasn't homesick; she was having panic attacks. (FYI: the medical doctor on staff assured us that he had observed her closely, and that there were no panic attacks.) Every call told a different tale; it was absolutely exhausting for all of us. According to Deidre, Anna had pretty quickly fallen into a routine of her own. The members of the corps would all show up on the field at the appointed time in the morning for a day of intense practice, and Anna would soon become ill and need to go to the clinic. The clinic happened to be staffed with a group of both male and female college-aged assistants whose job it was to wrap ankles, dispense Tylenol, put Band-Aids on boo-boos, you get it. Anna was in Heaven. She had them all to herself for the most part, and she seemed to like hanging out with the cool kids in the clinic. Remember, this was in the early days—corps had just started, and there were eleven weeks left. You see where this is going, right? I don't think I'm giving anything away to expand a little here. You see, the whole situation was then, and continues to be now, a mystery. I've probably read way more into it and should just chalk it up to good old-fashioned homesickness. Or just a complete change of heart. Who *doesn't* change their mind sometimes? It was really driving me nuts that she'd wanted this for so long and had worked so hard for it (and we had paid soooo much to make it happen) and now her attitude was as if she wanted to leave a movie because she'd lost interest in the plot. I just wasn't buying it; I needed details. I needed a reason, something or someone to blame. I was in Virginia, and my sixteen-year-old was in Iowa. I'd just finished drying the tears from putting her on the plane for her eleven-week adventure a few days ago, and now she wanted to come home.

Deidre called on Monday evening (seventy-two hours in) and told me that she'd issued an ultimatum to Anna, and she was sure that this would nip the issue in the bud. She told Anna that if she walked off the field one more time, she was going to be sent home. I knew right off the bat that this was the kiss of death for Anna's drum corps summer adventure. SCORE ONE for Anna! All she had to do was walk off the field as she'd done (several times) every day so far and she'd get to come home. Deidre had no idea what she'd done. I knew without a doubt that Anna would win this one, and that she'd be coming home.

Tuesday morning came, and Anna didn't walk off of the field—SHE JUST DIDN'T EVER STEP ONTO THE FIELD! And so, on Tuesday morning my phone rang, and on the other end was a very confused Deidre. Poor Deidre, who'd been so sure that she'd solved the problem, had played right into Anna's hands. Anna's a smart one, and she knew if Mom wouldn't let her come home then she'd find another way. Deidre threw the ball, and Anna knocked it out of the park. Now there was no choice, no going back. There were two hundred other corps members, and ultimatums had to be honored or chaos, the likes of which non-marching-band people cannot possibly understand, would ensue. Here's the thing: at this point we had NO idea why all this is going on. Anna had been obsessing about drum corps for over a year. Every move she'd made for months on end seemed to have one purpose, to get her closer to drum corps. And here we were, four days of Anna's *Dubuque, Iowa Heaven on Earth* and POOF! it was time to come home. There were no injustices to be remedied, no wrongs to be righted, nothing, nada. Just four days of back and forth *I want to come home, I don't want to come home, maybe I want to come home, I don't know what I want . . .* And so, after four painful, tearful days (my tears, not hers) we had a decision: Deidre was sending Anna home. At that point I had no choice but to make arrangements to get my girl back to Virginia.

And so, since this is my story, I'll tell you how I (mis)handled it. I got angry. Selfishly, childishly angry. That *so very sad* anger that words can't describe, that *I want to hit something, I want to cry, I want to run away* anger that proper mamas aren't supposed to feel. I was flooded with thoughts of the waste: wasted money, wasted time, wasted energy, wasted emotion. And fear. I was terrified for Anna. She'd spent the entire school year obsessing about marching drum with corps this summer; she'd talked about nothing else for months. How would she explain? What would she say? Senior year was on the horizon, and teenage kids can be so cruel (if you have teenage kids and you're offended by this, then I certainly wasn't referring to your kids—but you know the ones I mean). I could only imagine how painful it would be for her to go back to school and face the music (I know, that was a tasteless pun—but inappropriate humor sometimes helps keep the tears at bay).

Back to the point: how I handled Anna's return like a selfish, angry child. Step One was to get her a return flight home that day. The first one I could find was leaving the Dubuque airport in two hours and had two connections, not optimal but doable with some hustle. So, I called Anna and told her to pack quickly and tell Deidre she needed a ride. Could I have found a later flight, maybe even one without two connections? Sure. Could she pack up her special-sized suitcase with all of her special *eleven-weeks-of-supplies-for-four-days-of-drum-corps* and get to the airport to catch a flight that left in two hours? Sure, if she kicked it into high gear she sure could. And she did. She told us later that she even had time to catch up with all of her drum corps buddies and say a tearful, *I'll miss you so much* goodbye before she left. I found that part interesting since she was so intent on leaving, yet she was so sad to leave them behind. She certainly didn't seem to be running away from anyone or anything at drum corps, which she has insisted then and still insists now is the truth. Most everyone there treated her with kindness (I say most because there's a jerk in every crowd), and she made friends that she kept up with throughout the summer via her texting machine (Curt long ago gave that name to her cell phone since that's basically all she uses it for). She watched their performance and competition videos, celebrated their successes, shared the drama and trauma of their relationships, and even begged me to take her to see them all in person when they were near Virginia. She even sent care packages throughout the summer to her drum corps friends. I can honestly say that, as much as I'd like to blame her quick return home on something or someone at the corps, I just can't. There's nothing to indicate that anyone or anything there is to blame.

Step Two was to pout about the impact all of this would have on my upcoming summer adventures which included two vacations *with* Curt and definitely *without* kids (I've already confessed to being selfish and childish about this, so you can't call me out on that. I already own it). Best laid plans and all of that. We had booked two parents-only vacations that summer, with no travel insurance because I'm too cheap to buy it (can you even file an insurance claim for a missed vacation because your kid changed her mind and decided to come home from drum corps?), and now it looked like they weren't going to happen. Then there were the non-refundable one-way flights home from DCI in Indianapolis that we had paid for and wouldn't use; remember, Curt and I had planned to drive to DCI in August to meet Anna and fly home with her, after our no-kids-at-home summer. (Let's end the suspense here, because I know you're dying to find out what happened with all of this. We hired a fun, competent college grad student to move in with Anna [she had a blast; they made crochet necklaces and ate junk food and carbs] while we went on the two [guilt-ridden] vacations. And United Airlines got to sell our three seats to someone else. See, everybody won in the end.)

We (Curt and I) picked her up at the airport, and frankly that part is a blur. I think she cried, I think I cried, but we got in the car and went home. I don't remember a lot of conversation that night. I was partly relieved to have her back safe and sound, and partly furious at this whole screwed-up disaster.

If ever there was a parenting decision I've made that I've lived to regret EVERY SINGLE DAY since I made it, it was the decision to let Anna spend the summer (all whopping four days of it) marching drum corps. I own that decision. Anna pushed and pulled and begged and pleaded, but in the end, it was my decision. If memory serves, I'm the one who convinced Curt (remember, he's the practical, levelheaded parent in this family) that we should let her follow her dreams. I had watched my baby girl develop a passion for music that grew into a passion for drum corps, and come hell or high water, I was going to make sure she had the opportunity to follow her dream. She played trumpet, French horn, mellophone, and even drums which in my book made her quite the accomplished musician. I was incredibly proud of her for working so hard to get what she wanted and for accomplishing so much at such a young age. My heart told me to let her go to Iowa and live her dream; clearly, I should have let my brain have a say in the decision.

The next day it was time to get real, and basically the shit hit the fan for the first few days she was home. Here's the thing to understand here—there were still three weeks of school left, but she had already finished out the year. Seven teachers had allowed her to do the last few weeks of work in advance and to take her final exams before she left for drum corps. She couldn't go back to eleventh grade; there was nothing to do. Getting a summer job at this point likely meant working in fast food, which I was perfectly fine with, but there was not enough hell-no in hell-no when I told her to get the applications filled out. There was no way she was sitting on her ass all summer watching Netflix. Yes, those were my words. We were basically at an impasse. All of the jobs she wanted required you to be eighteen or over, and she was still sixteen. All of the places that hired sixteen-year-olds were places she absolutely refused to work. If you're reading this and thinking *you're the mom and you can make her get a job even if it's somewhere she doesn't want to work,* then clearly you've never been in a situation like this with a sixteen-year-old like this. Nobody could win here, and I knew it. We were at an impasse until I brilliantly (read sarcasm) realized that we had another option, an option way better than working fast food. SUMMER SCHOOL!! Here was my theory: she'd missed the last three weeks of school, seven teachers and a principal had gone out of their way to help her finish the school year three weeks early, and now here she sat with visions of Netflix and a comfy couch all summer. To me it was a no-brainer. She'd go to summer school. But here was the problem that she so quickly pointed out—she only needed two classes to graduate, English and Government. If she took one of those classes in the summer, then she had only one required class to take in her senior year. So, she came up with her own option; she'd take both English and Government in summer school, graduate early, and get on with her life.

ALL GROWN UP

Older parents whose kids are grown, or close to grown, almost always say the same thing to parents with younger kids: *They grow up so fast. You'll blink and they'll be all grown up and on their own, and then you'll miss them so much.* And most parents of younger kids, and by most parents I mean every parent I know except one (true story, I know exactly one person who does not buy into this) will smile politely at the older parent with the grown kids and *think* (not *say*, because that would be rude): *That's the biggest bunch of B.S. I've ever heard. I can't wait for them to grow up and get out on their own because they are wearing me out, and I need a break.*

But the older people with the grown kids are right, sort of. You miss them, but missing them is like childbirth. You forget the pain, or you minimize the pain, and you smile when you think about it. Nostalgia takes over and the memories become selective. Parents remember (hopefully) the good more than the bad (admit it, there's bound to be some bad). I smile when I remember Anna at ten years old throwing a fit because Christopher, Mallory, and Andrew were all "allowed" to do their own laundry. Only moms with a lot of kids truly realize how much laundry needs to get done with six people in the house, so I came up with the brilliant idea that each kid would begin to do their own laundry when they turned thirteen. The first three thought they were being punished, but not Anna. When she realized that she was the only one of the four not doing her own laundry, all hell broke loose. That was the day my very independent ten-year-old took over the washer and dryer. I don't miss those piles of laundry, but I sure do miss that ten-year-old.

CHAPTER 4

THE SUMMER

It's no use to go back to yesterday because I was a
different person then.

~ *Alice in Wonderland,* Lewis Carroll

Remember earlier when I said I secretly questioned whether
sending her to kindergarten on time was a mistake? Then that
other whopper when I let her go to Iowa? Well, now I secretly (not
a secret now) wonder if allowing Anna to graduate from high
school a year early was an equally horrendous mistake. Detecting a
pattern? But, I'm a logical person, and logical people know that you
can't go through life playing the *what-if* game.

The whole summer graduation thing was an adventure in itself.
It sounds pretty easy, actually. You decide what class(es) to take,
register, and go to school. Nope, not so easy. In our school district
summer school registration ended before the end of the school
year. Meaning that by the time Anna decided to pursue her most
excellent summer school adventure, we had approximately forty-

seven minutes to beat the deadline. Luckily, I never learned how to take no for an answer, so we got it done with three minutes to spare. There was one problem; Government class was full. She made it into the English class, but Government was a no-go. No room, no exceptions. But remember, *no* is not an acceptable answer in my world, and problem-solving is my middle name. Ask the right questions (or the same questions over and over and over until you've exhausted them) and you'll usually find a solution. Our solution was to take Government through the school system in the next county. It was an on-line class with just a few in-person meetings with the teacher, so my introverted soon-to-be-high-school-graduate didn't even have to meet new people. Not only did we have a solution, but we had a darn good one! (Side note: there was a drawback—Anna was really looking forward to the healthy debates that come with a room full of seventeen- and eighteen-year-olds discussing current events, the law and politics. Get her going on any of those topics and the introversion disappears in a flash. Fair warning: if you ever find yourself discussing any of those topics with her, you'd better bring your A-game, because she'll bring hers. She knows her facts, and she'll take you to the cleaners if you're not prepared.)

Twelfth grade summer English seemed straightforward. Drive fifteen minutes to one of the local high schools every Monday through Thursday for six weeks, stay there from 7:00 a.m. to 12:00 p.m., don't miss more than one day, don't be late more than three times, do your homework. Easy enough. This school wasn't Anna's home school, but no big deal. Summer school is only taught in a couple of locations, so chances were that she'd see some familiar faces from her high school. If not, then no big deal again. She's always been a great student and pretty much keeps to herself unless: 1) you approach her and strike up a conversation, or 2) you're a passionate champion for a cause, in which case she'll jump on board and be your best bud as you come together to right the wrongs of the world.

I didn't see summer school as a way for her to form any lasting friendships given the amount of work to be done in those six weeks. Finishing Government and senior English in six weeks is enough to keep anybody busy, and my goal was to keep Anna happy, focused, and productive, off of the couch and off of the television all day. This seemed like a means to that end. Making friends would be great, but quick bonding has never been her strong suit. So, when she came home one day during the first week and said that she'd made a friend I was thrilled, but a little surprised—it was just out of character for her. The new friend was Stephanie, also a seven-teen-year-old from a different high school. Over the six weeks I heard Stephanie's name quite a bit, and even suggested that Anna invite her over. Stephanie never showed up to visit, so I'm guessing Anna never actually invited her. No surprises there; it's never been Anna's nature to be proactive in new friendships.

Summer school ended quicker than you can say "forty-seven minutes left to register," and talk turned to community college. Anna was still sixteen (that September birthday again) and it made sense for her to take some classes that she'd enjoy (Sociology was one) and try to figure out where to go from there. My naïve assumption was that she'd go to community college for a year, get some classes under her belt, and start at a four-year school the next year with a few credits to carry over and a better idea of what she liked and what she didn't. She wanted a part-time job, and I was all over that. She ended up with two. Following her passion for animals, she ended up working as a pet sitter for a small local business and also at a pet store. She was able to go to school part time and also get her animal fix with all of the dogs, cats, and ponies she wanted.

By the end of August, it seemed like we'd left the drama/trauma of corps behind us and had found a new direction. Like I said, my goal for her was to be happy, focused, and productive. Two part-time jobs and a couple of classes kept her focused and productive, but the happiness part was clearly missing. It had been missing for a long time. Anna had been seeing a therapist for about eighteen months at this point, ever since she was about fourteen and a half. She saw Mona every week for the most part, and they were very close. Anna was very fond of her, trusted her, and had even asked Mona if she could call her from drum corps that summer if she needed to talk (Mona was very kind, so of course the answer was yes). She was anxious to get back to Mona when she came back home, but her summer school schedule and then her work schedule made it more difficult than it had been in the past, so she didn't see Mona every week; summer sessions were actually hit-or-miss. Honestly, I was a bit relieved that the therapy sessions were cut down. I liked Mona a lot, but I had the feeling that I was paying for a weekly playdate. The progress after eighteen months just wasn't there.

SEARCHING FOR KIKI

Anna was always fiercely independent, and if she wanted something, she just went for it. Just before her first birthday we bought a tiny cottage on the water in the quaint little village of Deltaville, Virginia. Hence, Anna grew up spending weekends on the water. She loved hanging out on the dock and looking for Kiki. Kiki was the name of each and every minnow that she managed to capture in her tiny net and then put in a bucket of river water until it was time to release Kiki and begin the search for the next one. She was adorable in her blue and yellow lifejacket, pacing the dock in her quest for Kiki. Anna had swimming lessons before she was two years old, and when she was finally old enough to participate I enrolled her in an intensive swim program that focused on one thing: teaching very young children to handle water mishaps and avoid drowning. They had the children jump into the pool, fully clothed including shoes (no lifejackets), and practice what they needed to do should they accidentally fall into the water. She thought that swimming in clothes and shoes was a blast.

One afternoon, not long after the swim program concluded, Anna was on the dock (lifejacket and sandals on–little feet can get splinters on the dock). Curt was with her, cleaning the boat as she conducted the daily Kiki ritual (no worries, she was never allowed near the water without an adult). Suddenly he heard a *splash* and looked up to see her in the water; she'd fallen in. Curt knew that he could get to her in seconds, so he decided to watch first and see how she'd handle it before he rushed to perform the water rescue. Just as he thought/hoped she'd do, Anna immediately gathered her wits and handled her little mishap all on her own. She swam to the end of the dock until she reached the back of the boat, held on to the boat as she grabbed the swim ladder, lowered the ladder into the water, and climbed up into the boat. And then? Then she walked around to the other side of the dock and continued the hunt for Kiki.

CHAPTER 5

THE THERAPIST

Go and love your children exactly as they are. And then, watch them become the truest and most wonderful versions of themselves. All they need . . . All anyone really needs . . . is to feel loved and appreciated for exactly who they are.

~ Wes Angelozzi

It's time for a little bit of background, so let's hold our place and talk about therapy for a bit, and then we'll get back to what happened at the end of the summer. Anna's first therapist was Mona. Mona was recommended to us by Anna's pediatrician when I told her that Anna needed help dealing with her unhappiness and extreme mood swings.

The first time we met with Mona (Anna and I saw her together for the first half of the session, then Anna went solo for the rest), Mona asked me a question that has been stuck in my brain since that day.

Mona: "What did you do for Anna when she was growing up to support her emotionally?"

Me (but only in my brain): "What the hell DIDN'T I do?!?"

Me (out of my mouth): "Well, (insert ridiculously blank stare here) I've always supported her emotionally. Her dad and I made sure she had all of the opportunities that we never had (ever heard that line before?). We supported everything she ever showed an interest in."

Mona: "But, (looking at me like a child who just doesn't understand the oh-so-simple question) how did you support her emotionally?"

Me (absolutely confused by now): "Well, I guess I should be more specific (looking at her with a *why-are-we-paying-for-this* look). When she wanted to do ballet when she was four, I made sure she got signed up. When she wanted to play soccer, or swim on swim team, or do karate, I made sure she was able to do that. When she started first grade and wanted to be a Girl Scout but none of the local troops had openings and none of the other parents with pouty-face little girls at the *let's join Girl Scouts* meeting would step up, I started a Girl Scout troop—I've been leading it now for nine years. When she wanted to join the marching band, I made sure she was able to do that, and I became a band mom so that I could be involved, too."

(At this point, I was feeling wildly accomplished as an emotionally supportive mom. I'm sure the look on my face radiated WINNER!)

Mona: "Maybe I'm not asking this the right way. It sounds like you're telling me about the things you gave her, that you paid for, but what have you done to support her emotionally?"

Me (wondering if there is a word for more confused than *absolutely confused*): "I'm pretty sure I just told you. Yes, we had to pay for those things in order for her to participate (you idiot, I thought to myself), but I was then and am now the one who makes sure she gets there and back on time, that she has what she needs to participate, that encourages her in everything she does, that helps out whenever they need a volunteer, I'm not sure how that's NOT emotional support."

Mona: "We'll get back to that question later. Maybe you can give it some thought after we finish today, and we can talk about it another time."

I was then dismissed to the waiting room so that the two of them could get started on their long journey of trying to unravel the damage done from my obvious inability to provide emotional support. Looking back, I realize my mistake. I totally forgot to tell her about my vegan chicken patty delivery before all the band events. That probably would have nipped the emotional support question in the bud. Hindsight (sigh).

On a serious note, I realized then that I had no answer for Mona's question, at least not the type of answer she wanted. That's one of the things that has haunted me for four years now. How could I be totally clueless in the parental emotional support zone? After four years it dawned on me that I clearly had no idea what parental emotional support really was, so I did what we all do when we're at a total and complete loss about something so important as your child's emotional well-being—you ask the great Google! Grab a seat and hold on when you google *parental emotional support*, because you're opening a can of worms.

The website ScienceDirect.com says that parental support has been defined as:

> Parental behaviors toward the child, such as praising,
> encouraging, and giving physical affection, which indicate
> to the child that he or she is accepted and loved.

Ok, I'm pretty sure I can deal with that. Anna certainly got plenty of the above. But wait, keep scrolling and there's more. On the flip side of the emotionally supportive parent is the emotionally unavailable parent.

From a blog post on PsychCentral.com: *What is an emotionally unavailable parent?*

Would you know what an emotionally detached and unavailable parent is? For most people who have endured an unstable, abusive, or **emotionally unavailable parent**, emotional detachment is an inability of the parent to meet their deepest needs, relate to them, or provides support and comfort when needed.

That one seems to miss the mark, disaster averted for now. But, just in case there's any confusion, there's a website called Clever Little Monkey that will guide you, step-by-step, on how to become an emotionally available parent.

1. Set aside regular times for the kids to talk to you.
2. Look them in the eyes when they talk to you.
3. Give your children the loving touch.
4. Keep track of important events and be sure to support them.

So, after being schooled via Google on parental emotional support I've come to two conclusions:

1. I still have no idea what I did right or did wrong or if I won the emotional support game or lost it big time.
2. I tried my hardest, I did my best, and I'm exhausted from all of this.

ANDY'S TOUR BUS

One day when Anna was thirteen-years old, I was at my office and she was at school. She called me from her cell phone (hiding in the bathroom since you couldn't use your cell phone at school). This was during the days of dark clothes and loud music with indecipherable words. Her favorite band was coming to another state, about two hours away from us, for a concert the next night, and we had tickets. I had agreed to take Anna and her friend to see the band, spend the night in a hotel room, and come home the next day. (I'd actually listened to their music and read the lyrics online, and while I wasn't a fan, I had to admit that their music was harmless.) Back to the phone call; it was an emergency.

It was the kind of emergency that only a thirteen-year-old girl can have, and only a former thirteen-year-old girl (like a mama) can understand. She was frantic. I could barely understand her between the frantic speech and the whispering and the acoustics in the bathroom. The emergency? The band's tour bus had been spotted parked at the shopping mall that was less than five miles from her school. Word travels fast, and I think the word came from her BFF who lived in the apartments adjacent to the shopping mall and who conveniently happened to be skipping school that day and spotted the bus. A few text messages later and she had confirmation.

Anna was a basket case. She had to get to that bus, and she needed me to leave work NOW. After listing all of the reasons why I couldn't possibly leave, I caved. I called the school, made up some excuse for why I needed to pick her up early, and off we went to meet the school-skipping BFF and sit in a parking lot staring at an empty bus. We were there for hours. At one point we walked up to the bus and we actually knocked on the door. Empty bus. (No, I was not going to let any of us go into the bus. Plus, we were in broad daylight with tons of people and traffic around us, so we were in a very safe environment.) Then we saw a few guys in the band walk across the parking lot, go into the bus, and come out with a soccer ball. Now we were sitting in a parking lot watching a couple of band-guys play soccer.

I was actually sitting in the car, by now feeling like a crazy person, while the two star-struck young ladies sat on the grass and stared at the soccer players. They gathered up the courage to walk over (with me) to the soccer players and ask when they might have a chance to see Andy, their favorite band-guy. Neither guy knew Andy's whereabouts or when he'd be back, so we continued to wait. At one point the girls decided that Andy was probably hungry after being on the road, so logically that meant he'd be in a nearby restaurant. He had no choice but to walk since the massive tour bus was still there right in front of us next to the soccer players.

So next I drove the girls around so that they could peek in the windows of every restaurant within walking distance. We looked like freaks. Still no Andy, so back to park the car across from the tour bus and wait. And then it happened, the stars aligned, and our mission was accomplished—Andy walked across the parking lot and into the bus. Next came a frantic meltdown as each girl begged the other to go and knock on the door of the bus. I'd finally had enough, so I told them that we were all three going to knock together. And we did. And Andy answered the door to the bus. And the girls froze; they couldn't move, they couldn't speak. I, on the other hand, had plenty to say, which embarrassed the crap out of the two girls. I told Andy how much the girls loved his music and how we had seen them in concert a few months ago and how we were going to see him again the next night. Anna and the BFF turned fifty shades of red. What's a mama to do when she's embarrassed two teenage girls beyond belief? She pulls out the cell phone and lines everyone up for a pose by the bus to take photos. I have the photos to prove it.

You can't make this stuff up, can you? Life is sometimes stranger than fiction.

CHAPTER 6
THE AFTER

Love isn't a state of perfect caring. It is an active noun like struggle. To love someone is to strive to accept that person exactly the way he or she is, here and now.

~ Fred "Mr." Rogers

———————————

So back to the end of summer, after drum corps, after summer school, after the calm but before the storm.

Remember Stephanie, from summer school senior English? Well, Stephanie's name hadn't been mentioned much since midway through summer school. Now we're at the end of August, at what would have been the beginning of Anna's senior year with band practice and all of its trauma and glory, but was now her summer of graduation and new beginnings. Anna was fully immersed in her part-time jobs and had registered for psychology and sociology at the one of the local community colleges. Everything seemed to be on an even keel, and I was hoping for new friends (for Anna) with her new beginning. She could leave the past behind and be whatever she wanted to be. The world was her oyster. The sky was the limit. More clichés; forgive me. Now, when I say that she could be whatever she wanted to be, I meant an artist, or a lawyer, or maybe a dermatologist. But, alas, it was not to be so simple.

Anna, it turns out, wanted to be a guy.

So, what has that to do with Stephanie? Stephanie, as it happens, actually went by the name *Stephan*, and Stephan was/is a transgender male, AFAB (assigned female at birth), born a female and identifying as a male. And that summer, the summer after, Anna announced that she, too, was a transgender male, AFAB, born a female and identifying as a male. Oh, and an interesting little fun fact here: she decided to tell me all of this as I'm driving down a winding country road with her riding shotgun.

I must admit, throughout the summer, the after, I'd had an inkling that something was up. Truth? I had a feeling that Anna was a lesbian. And I was totally cool with that. Seriously. Curt and I had even talked about it, the *maybe Anna is a lesbian* part. I'm not a lesbian, but I'm not homophobic, either. Homosexuality has become a societal norm, the stigma of years past just isn't there anymore (again, my perspective here). I have friends who are homosexual, but in my brain they're simply friends, not homosexual friends. But to have your cute-as-a-button almost seventeen-year-old daughter tell you she's transgender, that she should have been born a male, that her whole life up to this point has been like living a lie, is a shock. She wanted us to start calling her *Lucas*. Oh, and if we could use male pronouns immediately (he, him, his), that would be great.

Now, I love my children, all of them. And this one, number four, Anna (Lucas?), the one who would have been called *Tessa*, has always been challenging—taking me over bumps that I never saw coming. But this was a boulder, not a bump. Thinking your child is homosexual is one thing (kind of an *ok, it is what it is, no big deal* thing), but having your child tell you that they're a different gender is . . . well, WTF?!?

Back to the car ride (winding road, Anna/Lucas riding shotgun and dropping boulders as we go along our merry way). After she dropped that one on me I had only a few words, and they were something close to this: "No you're not, and what does that even mean?" And so, Anna/Lucas explained:

- Anna/Lucas had always felt like a male.
- Anna/Lucas was always afraid to tell us for fear of our reaction. She/he was convinced that Curt and I would kick her/him out of the house. In fact, she/he had already spoken with her friend, Krystal, about coming to live with Krystal's family should we tell her/him to leave the house.
- The people at the pet store where she/he worked already knew and were calling her/him Lucas.
- The lady who owned the pet sitting service where she also worked already knew and had been a great source of comfort and acceptance.
- Another friend's mom knew, and that mom was also a great source of comfort and acceptance and had even ordered a binder for Anna/Lucas to wear to bind her/his chest. (I'm still a little sticky on that one; not sure I'd have done the same had I been in that mom's shoes. But, alas, this is a no judgement venue, so it is what it is.)

Let's just say that the rest of the car ride was weird. I was given the dubious honor of relaying all of this to Curt. The rest of the day was pretty much a blur.

You can imagine (or maybe you can't) the barrage of emotions at that point (my emotions, remember this is my tale). How did this happen? When did this happen? What did this mean? What in the hell had I paid Mona for? This was a pretty big deal, and you mean to tell me that a therapist hadn't caught onto this in eighteen months of weekly sessions? Or had she caught on and just not felt the need to tell me (I know, patient confidentiality and all of that, even at age sixteen).

We spent the weekend catching our breath (the car ride with the winding roads had been a trip to the river for the weekend). It was too much; it was overwhelming–the questions, the confusion, the emotions. Then back to Mona—remember, Mona sessions had been sort of hit-or-miss with summer school and two part-time jobs. By this time Anna/Lucas was driving herself/himself pretty much everywhere, including therapy. But this time we went together—I needed it as much as she/he did.

I'd like to pause here and make a proclamation. Going forward, at least for a couple of chapters, I'm going to refer to Anna as Anna (not Lucas), and I'm going to use female pronouns (she, her, hers). Before you label me an unsupportive hater, here me out: there is a change coming, so having you get accustomed to Lucas is a waste of your time and energy. Keep reading; you'll get it soon enough.

Remember the part a few paragraphs back when Anna told me she was transgender, and I ever so inappropriately proclaimed, "No you're not . . ."? Well, my hope was that Mona could help fix that little blunder of mine. So, off we go to see Mona. Anna obviously had hopes that Mona would straighten me out, and I had hopes that Mona would be the one to act like a grown-up in this situation (and I hoped that she would straighten Anna out, truth be told).

Neither one of us got what we wanted. We walked in, sat down on the under-stuffed, 1972 vintage couch, told Mona our latest news (you're with me, right—the news is the part about Anna being transgender) and both waited for Mona to take care of this situation once and for all. Anna and I were both ready for the words of wisdom that we were sure would come from Mona's mouth. Mona listened to both of us, took it all in, opened her mouth and said to Anna, "No you're not . . ." Where have you heard that before?!?

As much as I wanted to "win" by having Mona affirm my position, having her spit out the same words I did a few days earlier wasn't what I considered to be a good thing. And if I thought it wasn't a good thing, Anna thought it was a train wreck. There are no words that Mona could have uttered that would have been worse than those. I know she didn't mean for it to come out that way; she's a therapist but she's human. She was just as shocked as I was when I heard it for the first time. So, Mona recovered, a little, and proceeded to explain why she just didn't buy this. She told Anna that, although she hadn't seen her much over the past few months, she'd seen her weekly for eighteen months until just about three months ago. She pointed out that at no point over those eighteen months had Anna shown any signs or made mention of gender dysphoria, being transgender, etc. I explained that this was my point exactly, but my time frame was a little longer; over the span of seventeen years I'd seen no signs. I'd been completely blindsided by this whole thing.

Anna insisted differently. She claimed that she had mentioned this to Mona (the look on Mona's face told a different story). She said that I'd just missed the signs at home. Remember when she was in preschool and wanted to get a haircut like Daddy? No, frankly I didn't remember that. But it would not have surprised me. She worshiped her Daddy, to the point that if anyone in the family sat next to him other than her (dinner table, watching television, church, whatever) she cried like her world had ended. He was her everything when she was little. That was about the best example of gender dysphoria she could come up with at the time, but she insisted that she'd known she was male since she was in preschool. And Mona just wasn't buying it. We ended the session as we had so many times before, me in the waiting room and Anna finishing up whatever she was finishing up with Mona. But this time when she came out to go home it was different. She was done with Mona. No more Mona, no way no how. Anna had made another appointment, but that was only to tell Mona what she thought of her and to tell her she was never coming back.

BEFORE WAS NORMAL

Anna, when she was Anna, once said to me, "Normal is a setting on the dryer." At the time I thought this to be an odd comment coming from a pre-teen, but pre-teens are odd creatures anyway. I think that maybe I get it now, the dryer comment. I haven't felt normal since the car ride on the winding road. Normalcy went out of the window that day, and I doubt it will return. No matter how tolerant/progressive/accepting you are, the normal life that my family lived up until that day is gone. People often refer to the "new normal." I also used to refer to the "new normal," but I'm not sure there is such a thing anymore. There's before and after. Before was normal for me. After is anything but normal. After is a struggle, a fog, a constant state of confusion. After is walking on eggshells, afraid that the wrong name will slip out of my mouth, or, even worse, the wrong pronoun. After is not normal.

CHAPTER 7

THE HAMMER

To someone with a hammer, everything looks like a nail.

~ Mark Twain

If you've ever tried to navigate the world of mental health, especially the world of childhood/teen mental health, then you know that it's no easy task. Anna had seen Mona for months, and suddenly Mona was out of the picture. No more Mona meant no more therapy, which meant that we needed to find a replacement pretty quickly. Anna was clearly going through things in her life that needed more help than I could possibly begin to give.

Fun fact about Anna: she's a prolific researcher. With Mona kicked to the curb, it was time for Anna to find a replacement. Anna WANTED a replacement for Mona. She was always willing to tell her story to anyone who would listen, and having a therapist meant that Anna had her own captive audience each and every week for a whole hour. After talking to a few people she knew in the LGBTQ world and doing her own research (Google really is amazing, isn't it), Anna found Debra.

Debra's claim to fame was her specialty in working with young adults in the transgender world. She's a licensed clinical psychologist, a Ph.D., so we were upping our game; Mona was a LCSW, a licensed clinical social worker. Debra's goal, had you asked her (and I did), was to help young people with gender dysphoria self-discover and determine their true path in life. This was her specialty, her passion, and her life's work. She had spent twenty-plus years working with thousands of young people who struggled with gender dysphoria. FYI, gender dysphoria is the mental distress felt by a person whose body does not match their gender identity. I felt like we were onto something. Finally, someone who would be able to help us sort this whole thing out so that I could have my Anna back and life as we knew it *before* would return.

Debra explained that she'd need between three and five sessions with Anna—Debra called her Lucas—to get this whole situation sorted out, and then she could make an assessment as to how we should proceed. These sessions were a combo package of seeing Anna individually and conducting family therapy (Anna, Curt, and me). The mission, according to Debra, was to first help Anna determine if she was, indeed, transgender or to figure out if there was something else going on. What we knew for sure was that Anna was unhappy and depressed (two very different emotions). I realize now how naïve I was then, but when you're blinded by hope you'll grab on to anything with a vengeance. And I was so hopeful and so blinded.

Neither Mona nor Debra were medical doctors, so they obviously couldn't prescribe medication. However, both therapists had urged us to seek some help for Anna from a medical doctor because both felt strongly that Anna needed prescription medications to deal with depression. The residuals from that depression included anger, belligerence and explosive reactions to anything and everything that came across her radar that she didn't like or didn't agree with (but only at home, as we were the sole beneficiary of Anna's rage). Hence, Anna was also seeing Dr. Davidson, a medical doctor (psychiatrist) to get those prescriptions. You'll hear more about Dr. Davidson later.

In the meantime, life at home was pretty much hell. I'll stop here and tell you the two things that got me through then and continue to get me through now: my faith and a strong marriage. When you're going through this hell on earth that has become your family life, there are only two people who can possibly understand —one is God, and the other is the person who's holding your hand and walking through it with you.

The three to five sessions with Debra turned into six or eight, and things at home had gone from bad to worse. Here's an email exchange between me and Debra that I think sums it up nicely:

Me: "During our first meeting you indicated that you would likely meet with Anna individually three to five times. I believe we are at that point and wonder about our direction going forward. Anna has become increasingly difficult and belligerent. She argues more than ever—screaming, name calling (calling us stupid, ignorant, etc). Dr. Davidson has increased her Prozac to twenty milligrams without an improvement that we can see.

Anna does have the capability to be pleasant, but only when you are agreeing with her one hundred percent. If you disagree with her about anything at all she launches into a screaming tirade, accusing you of not listening to anything she says. It is really getting to be quite ridiculous. She acts more like a four-year-old than a seventeen-year-old.

Curt and I do not see where she is making any progress. This whole situation seems to be giving her just more and more reason to argue and pick fights. Knowing where we all stand, is there a compelling reason for her to continue weekly sessions? What is the endgame? It appears that we are at a standstill until she turns eighteen."

(As with most teenagers, Anna saw age eighteen as the magic

bullet to solve all of life's problems, and she was quite vocal about how everything would be fine as soon as she turned eighteen. If you have teenagers, or if you've even been a teenager, then you definitely get it.)

Debra: "Hi Patti . . . you are right in that we have already completed the initial tentative schedule of several individual sessions plus a parent follow-up. I see current goals as being about 1) managing dysphoria and 2) future planning. I do feel as though Anna is experiencing significant distress and would benefit from continuing therapy, but obviously, that is a family decision."

Maybe it's just me, but that seemed like a non-answer. I followed with this:

Me: "Curt and I have agreed to allow Anna to continue with the sessions with the expectation that Anna will use these sessions productively in an effort to be a more amicable member of the family/household. If we don't see that she is working toward improvement soon then we will reassess."

Debra: "Okay, sounds good. And I agree that everyone in the household should be a 'good citizen' of that household."

Certainly good to hear that we were on the same page. I thought/hoped we were on the same page, but exactly what page were we on? Were we on the page where we all want to help Anna sort through this, or were we on the page where Debra was telling us she was trying to help Anna sort through all of this but was really just taking Anna on a stroll down the transgender highway? Curt stepped in a couple of days later with his own question. Remember, Debra's professional mission in life, her passion, was to help youth suffering with gender dysphoria find their true path through a combination of therapy and self-discovery.

Curt: "Debra, I was talking with Patti this morning and I had a question. What percentage of youth, like Anna, do you counsel that actually discover they are not transgender?"

Debra: "Hi Curt . . . to my knowledge, none of the several hundred youth I've counseled over the years who have asserted a trans identity have decided they're not transgender, though I've worked with some young children whose parents thought their children were trans and they ended up not being trans. I have had a few youths who have shifted from a binary trans identity to a non-binary identity, and vice versa. (Three or four, maybe.) Of course, I don't know what happens with youth when I no longer see them."

My practical, *tell it like it is* husband then came up with the perfect analogy. If Debra was a hammer, then everyone she sees was a nail. He hit it right on the head (useless pun again, sorry this time).

Debra was clearly focused on gender transition, which is exactly what it sounds like: socially, legally, and/or medically changing how you present yourself to reflect your gender identity. Do you know what the opposite of gender transition is? If you guessed *detransition* then you got it! Dying to know more? Let's let Wikipedia explain:

> **Detransition** is the cessation or reversal of
> a transgender identification or gender transition, whether
> by social, legal, or medical means. It is estimated that
> detransitioners range from less than one percent to as many
> as eight percent of individuals who start transition. Some
> individuals detransition on a temporary basis. **Desistance** is
> a related term used to describe the cessation of transgender
> identity or gender dysphoria and has a higher occurrence.

The logical question here is: Where's the research on *detransition*? Wiki to the rescue, again (everything in bold is my emphasis):

> *Direct, formal research of detransition is lacking. Professional*
> *interest in the phenomenon has been met with contention.*
> *Detransitioners (persons who detransition) have similarly experi-*
> *enced controversy and struggle.*
> *Like transition, detransition is not a single event. Methods of*
> *detransitioning can vary greatly among individuals, and can*
> *involve changes to one's gender expression, social identity, legal*

identity documents, and/or anatomy. Those who undertake detransition are known as detransitioners. Detransition is commonly associated with transition regret, but regret and detransition do not always coincide.

Formal studies of detransition have been few in number, of disputed quality, and politically controversial. Frequency estimates for detransition and desistance vary greatly, with notable differences in terminology and methodology. Detransition is more common in the earlier stages of transition, particularly before surgeries. A 2018 survey of WPATH (World Professional Association for Transgender Health) surgeons found that approximately 0.3% of patients who underwent transition-related surgery later requested detransition-related surgical care. The 2015 U.S. Transgender Survey found that 8% of respondents who had transitioned reported having ever detransitioned, and 62% of that group had later returned to living in a transgender role.

What about transgender adolescents, you may ask?

Desistance in gender dysphoric adolescents may be higher. A 2008 study found 61% desisted from their transgender identity before reaching the age of twenty-nine, and a 2013 study found 63% desisted before age twenty. A 2019 clinical assessment found that 9.4% of patients with adolescent-emerging gender dysphoria ceased wishing to pursue medical interventions and/or no longer felt that their gender identity was incongruent with their biological sex within an eighteen-month period.

A 2017 study suggested detransition rates are growing. A 2003 German study found evidence for an increase in the number of demands for detransition, **blaming poor practice on the part of "well-meaning but certainly not unproblematic" clinicians who —contrary to international best practices—assumed that transitioning as quickly as possible should be the only correct course of action.** Surgeon Miroslav Djordjevic and psychotherapist

*James Caspian have reported that demand for surgical reversal of
the physical effects of medical transition has been on the rise.*

**Detransitioners have commonly cited trauma, isolation, dissoci-
ation, inadequate mental healthcare, and social pressure as
motivations for pursuing transition. Informed consent and affirmation of self-diagnosis (both newer but increasingly employed
models for transgender healthcare) have been criticized for
failing to meet the needs of those who eventually detransition.
Among eventual detransitioners, the progression of transition
has been found to magnify, rather than remedy, gender
dysphoria. Sufferers may fixate on passing (being perceived as
their preferred gender), leading them to pursue ever further steps
in medical transition.**

*Motives for detransitioning commonly include financial barriers
to transition, social rejection in transition, depression or suici-
dality due to transition, and discomfort with sexual characteristics developed during transition. Additional motives include
concern for lack of data on long-term effects of hormone replacement therapy, concern for loss of fertility, complications from
surgery, and changes in gender identity. Some people detransition
on a temporary basis, in order to accomplish a particular aim,
such as having biologically related children, or until barriers to
transition have been resolved or removed. Transgender elders
may also detransition out of concern for whether they can receive
adequate or respectful care in later life.*

After two months of weekly sessions with Debra we called it
quits. Anna needed someone to help her navigate through this
gender dysphoria and possible gender transition, but first she
needed to figure out who she really was. I needed someone to guide
Anna to her fork in the road so that she could figure out which path
to take. There were clearly no forks in Debra's road; it was a straight
path down the transgender highway.

Don't get me wrong, I'm a firm believer in therapy. I know that there are many wonderful therapists out there, both Ph.D.s and medical doctors, whose number one priority is to help their patients. Our challenge was finding one who was taking new patients without a nine month wait list.

SOMEONE TO LISTEN

You already know I'm Catholic. Catholics have lots of favorites: favorite saint, favorite sacrament, favorite seat at Mass (and God help the poor soul who unknowingly sits in it). I, like so many other brother/sister Catholics, have a favorite priest, Father John. He passed away a few years ago, but he will forever be my favorite. He is irreplaceable, and I miss him every day. He was wise, dynamic, and dramatic. And he would have LOVED holding my hand through this journey of transgender confusion; just being part of the whole situation would have thrilled him to no end. He'd known Anna since before she was born, and he'd been a significant presence in our family for over twenty years. This transgender thing would have been just up his alley. He would have called me out every time I screwed up (which would have been often). He would have listened, but he would never have "taken sides." BUT if forced to "take sides" I'm convinced that he would have sided with Anna. He'd have told me to put my big-girl pants on and let her journey through life as she saw fit. He'd tell me that she'd figure it out. He'd tell me that I had raised her as I saw fit, and now it was her turn to live her life as she saw fit. He'd tell me to get over myself because it was my turn to be a spectator in the story of her life, and that she'd let me know when it was time to be a player again. He'd tell me that everything really would be okay. And, he'd mean it.

John may be gone, but the John-isms will never go away. The John-ism that keeps calling to me is the *Hole in the Soul*. That's what he named that feeling that consumes you, that won't go away. That feeling that *if only* . . . If only I could change it. If only I could control it. If only THEY could see it the way I see it. If only, if only, if only. The *Hole in the Soul* is that thing that you absolutely cannot change, you know you can't change it, you can't fix it, but you just can't figure out how to make peace with it either. If he were here, he'd tell me that Anna's transgender journey was my *Hole in the Soul*, and I need to find a way to make peace with it. He would tell me what I already know; that God loves my number four whether she calls herself Anna or Lucas.

CHAPTER 8

THE PUPPY

When your children are teenagers it's important to have a dog so
that someone in the house is happy to see you.

~ Nora Ephron

Let's regroup—summer school is over, high school graduation has
happened (no gown, no ceremony, but we did have a party to celebrate), the two part-time jobs are in full swing, and Anna's taking a
few classes at the community college. And she's as unhappy as I've
ever seen her. One therapist (Mona) was kicked to the curb (by
Anna) for not believing that Anna was transgender and suggesting
that we dive deeper and find out if there was something else going
on. Another therapist (Debra) was dismissed (by me) for refusing to
even consider that: 1) Anna MIGHT NOT be transgender and, 2)
that we needed to dive deeper and find out if there was something
else going on.

They're calling her Lucas at work; we're calling her Anna at
home (and honestly most of the time at this point I just avoided

using a name at all). She wants us to use male pronouns, to accept the fact that Anna was gone, and Lucas was here. She began to talk about a legal name change as soon as she turned eighteen (at this point she's barely seventeen). I even offered to take her to the county courthouse to file the papers, smug and certain that she'd never actually go through with it. I reminded her that a name change is a big deal, and that she needs to be one hundred percent sure that the name she takes is the one she wants. Then she surprised me. She presented me and Curt with a list of about seven names, first and middle, and she asked us to vote on them. She liked all of them, was having a hard time deciding, and thought that we'd like some input into her new name. (What I actually wanted at this point was to wake up and realize that for once I'd been sleeping and this was all a bad dream.) We cast our vote for Tristan Blaine. She liked it, we liked it, so Anna Marie was now to be called Tristan Blaine. Lucas was out.

Somehow this managed to bring me a little comfort. Tristan sounded almost androgynous, so I could deal with it a little better than Lucas. Nothing legal at this point, but I agreed to try calling her Tristan. But, the he/him/his? I just wasn't there. It's hard; it was hard then and it's hard now. I became a pronoun-less mama when Anna became Tristan. My mouth WILL NOT let the he/him/his come out when I'm talking about my daughter. Do I try with the pronouns? I'd be lying if I said *yes*, because I don't try. I don't because I can't. It seems ridiculous to me that I would refer to her as a male. I might as well call Mallory *he* and Christopher and Andrew *she*. That makes as much sense to me as calling Anna *he*. My four children have been a constant source of joy and tears (alternating) for more than half of my life; one minute you're bursting with pride at the wonder of them and the next minute you want to go hide in a closet and never come out. Do you want to know one of my favorite things as a mama of four? It's silly, but here goes. It's when someone says, "Oh, do you have boys or girls?" And I say, "Two of each, boy girl boy girl." Invariably they respond with, "How perfect!" And, yes, it's perfect. Boy girl boy girl.

If you've walked in my shoes and it was a piece of cake for you to flip the switch and go from having a daughter one day to having a son the next, then that's awesome. That means you may have avoided the torment that has consumed my thoughts for so long now, and that has impacted every part of my life each and every day since that car ride down the winding road. I hate that road now. Every time I drive it I see my sweet daughter with her too-tight jeans, t-shirt cut a little too low, bleached blonde hair, and eyeliner, sitting next to me and telling me she's not, in fact, a girl at all.

At this point we have an unhappy, depressed seventeen-year-old who is trying to navigate life as a different gender, with a different name, and with little social interaction other than what she gets at work or at school (she was taking a few classes at a local community college). She gets frustrated when customers at the pet store call her *ma'am*, but she certainly didn't look like a *sir*. She's not making friends at school, but at this point I totally blame Stephanie for our latest predicament, so I think making friends at school is definitely overrated.

I was absolutely no help at this point. I was in unchartered waters and felt like I was sinking fast. Kids, even seventeen-year-olds, so often expect their parents to have all of the answers, to fix everything or at least to have a lifeboat to offer when they start to sink. I had no answers, no fixes, and not even a buoy ring to toss out, much less a lifeboat.

So, what's a control-freak mama to do when she's lost control and cannot find a way to help her kid? That's easy—she gets the kid a puppy!! Yes, a puppy. A puppy would fix everything, right? A puppy would give Tristan (trying to get the hang of the new name) someone to love and care for. They could bond; they could snuggle. A puppy would be fun. A puppy would make Tristan happy. A puppy would heal the depression. We would all love the puppy. We would spend our evenings at home playing with the puppy and laughing at the puppy. We'd be so busy having fun with the puppy that we wouldn't have any time to argue; who can argue when you're so busy laughing at the adorable puppy? Puppies really do fix everything!!

(Time for a side note: at the time all of this was happening we had a wonderful older pup named Princess. Princess was THE best dog there ever was, I'm convinced of it. She was loved more than I can say. However, Princess was old. And lazy. She slept all day and was definitely not a snuggler. We needed to up our canine game and add another one that could step in and fix everything for us faster than you could scream *"QUICK, TAKE HER OUTSIDE, SHE'S PEEING ON THE FLOOR AGAIN!"*)

My puppy plan had just the tiniest little hiccup. Anna (before she became Tristan) had been singing the *I Want a Puppy Song* for a while, and Curt was having absolutely no part of it. As far as he was concerned Princess was the final chapter in our dog book. He had refused to even consider a puppy. I, on the other hand, have always been a sucker for a puppy, so Curt was used to me siding with Anna every time she found another puppy that she wanted to bring home (she was working in a pet store, so there was always a puppy to bring home). Anna would show us a picture of an adorable pup, I'd point out how adorable it was, and Curt would tell me that my next husband and I could have as many puppies as we wanted (somehow he thought this was funny). His *no puppy* stance was quite firm, until it wasn't. It all changed when Anna became Tristan. Desperate times called for desperate measures, and Curt finally saw the logic in adding a puppy to our mixed-up mix.

We (Curt, Tristan, and I finally agreeing on something) chose a tiny, two-pound ball of white fluff that Tristan named Calypso. That name lasted about seven minutes since Tristan and I both realized that Calypso is a great name for a large, regal dog (maybe a Great Dane or a Siberian Husky) but not so much for a tiny fluff ball who'll only grow into a slightly less tiny fluff ball. (FYI, she's a whopping ten pounds at age two.) Calypso was shortened to Caly, and our short-term mission was accomplished. Caly was (and still is) a bundle of love and joy wrapped up in a white fluffy jacket. And while I don't advocate answering all of life's problems with a puppy, she certainly helped us as we were trying to navigate around a pretty big boulder in our family road. Adding a puppy is almost like adding a toddler: feeding schedules, nap times, potty training. Caly made us laugh and kept us busy. She also distracted us from the angst that was our lives; she gave us something else to focus on rather than our constant disagreements about gender and pronouns. Caly didn't solve our problems, but she sure did (and continues to) give us a reason to smile as we struggle. Princess (God rest her wonderful soul) even learned to tolerate Caly.

Pretty soon, however, it was obvious that adding Caly to our family was like putting a Band-Aid on a hemorrhage. She gave us a common ground, a neutral territory. Caly was goofy and happy, and she always made you smile. But our family was hemorrhaging pain of a unique sort, and puppy love can't take that away. We had the pain of a child who was trying to leave her whole identity behind and struggling to find her place in her new world. We had the pain of a mom who just wanted the whole situation to go away, who wanted to put her head in the sand so she didn't have to deal with it. I didn't want to learn about correct pronouns, and binders, and gender dysphoria, and name changes. I hadn't signed up for any of this. I wanted my daughter back. I think that maybe this whole situation might have been easier to process had Tristan been happy, but she just wasn't.

To make matters worse, I just flat out didn't believe any of it. I did not believe for one second that Tristan, my Anna Marie, was transgender. But, at the same time, I didn't believe that Tristan was lying (who would lie about that?). So, how could I not believe her and yet be convinced she wasn't lying? Beats me. I didn't know Tristan. I knew Anna, and Anna was as honest as they come. So now there was an even bigger question to lose sleep over; what the hell is REALLY going on here? (Spoiler alert: I still don't have the answer to that.)

Here's what I KNEW, in a nutshell:

• Anna left Virginia as Anna.
• Anna came back from Iowa as Anna.
• Anna started summer school as Anna.
• Anna finished summer school as Lucas, proclaiming to be transgender, after making a friend in summer school who just happened to be transgender.
• Anna/Lucas was now going by Tristan Blaine.
• Anna's BFF therapist who'd seen her fifty plus times was totally blindsided by all of this.
• Anna's parents, siblings, and grandparents were totally blindsided by all of this.
• Anna was unhappy and depressed.

And here's what I THOUGHT:

• Anna put way too much pressure on herself over this drum corps thing and was embarrassed at the outcome.
• Anna's self-esteem was practically nonexistent; it was low before Iowa and pretty much gone now.
• Anna didn't like who she was (Anna, before Lucas or Tristan even came into the picture).
• Anna wanted to be anyone BUT Anna when she got back from her four-day adventure in Iowa.
• Anna thought that being Lucas/Tristan was the answer to all of the above.

Here we were, about three months into this transgender world, and I was so lost and confused that there's no way I could help my child—my smart, funny, beautiful little girl who was still smart, funny, and beautiful but not my little girl anymore.

If only we could really answer all of life's problems with a puppy.

YOU JUST KNOW

Did you ever get a new car and think to yourself, *this is such a cool car, I've never seen another one this color.* Then suddenly everywhere you look there are cars in that exact same cool color. Well, that's sort of the analogy of my life since we entered the ranks of *Family with a Transgender Member.* I kid you not, suddenly my world is filled with transgender persons.

There was the transgender female (AMAB) flight attendant who was super friendly and absolutely delightful. Next came the chatty transgender male (AFAB) passenger on the train who was happy to share navigational tips with me since I clearly had tourist stamped on my forehead. Then came the transgender male (AFAB) fast food worker with a big smile and a bigger basket of fries. Yes, those are a few examples of the many transgender folks that have crossed my path since Tristan's announcement. How, you may ask, do I know they're transgender? Well, you just know. As hard as they try, sometimes (not always, but sometimes) you can just tell. And what's the point of sharing my encounters with these ladies and gentlemen, anyway? The point is this: my brief encounter with each told me that they all have one thing in common. They all seem quite comfortable in their current skin. Stay with me, the real point is coming.

I'm clearly struggling with Tristan's transgender identity, no shocker there. I often ask myself what would make it easier to accept all of this. And I think I know the answer. I think I could more easily accept Tristan's transgender identity if I believed one hundred percent that she was happy in her new world. And I don't believe it, not for a minute. She projects anything but a person who is happy with who they are. She's restless, a rebel with a cause— any cause. Her life (or what she shares with me) seems to be an endless series of this protest to that rally and back again. Transgender rights? She'll march with you. Gun control? Where does she sign up? Civil unrest in some foreign nation whose name I can't even pronounce? Thank goodness she lives close enough to make it to Washington D.C. and back in a day to join the rally. So, the point is this: she's still very much trying to figure out who she is, and she doesn't appear any happier as Tristan than she was as Anna. And that in itself absolutely breaks my heart.

CHAPTER 9

THE FLAGS

See, people come into your life for a reason. They might not know
it themselves, why. You might not know it. But there's a reason.
There has to be.

~ Joyce Carol Oates

At this point in our journey Tristan was, understandably, furious
that I still questioned her male identity. This was right in the
middle of the Lucas to Tristan transition, too.

It wasn't just Curt and me who were completely blindsided by
the disappearance of Anna Marie and the appearance of Tristan
Blaine. Anna's three older siblings were caught off guard as well,
although their reactions were each different.

The older two, Christopher and Mallory, drew a pretty hard line
in the sand—they just flat out didn't buy it. Christopher's stance
was pretty hard-core—"I don't believe it, this is bullshit, I'm not
calling her Lucas or Tristan, or whatever the hell she calls herself."
Christopher looked at Tristan and saw Anna, his baby sister. After

all, she still looked like Anna. He was ten years older, and he saw the little girl that he had cradled in his arms when she was a baby. He saw the little sister who always wanted to tag along behind him and his friends, who said that Chris' best friend was her boyfriend, and said that she was going to marry him when she grew up. The thought of that little cutie pie suddenly announcing that she was a male was really more than he could handle, and the thought of it just made him angry.

Mallory didn't buy it either, but she tried to approach the situation with more understanding. She thought that she should spend more time with Anna, and she made a real effort to call her Tristan. (Mallory was the only one of the four who had moved out of town; she lived two hours away, so spending more time together wasn't easy.) Mallory thought that she should become more of a friend so that Tristan would have someone she could talk to. She was eight years older, and when she thought of Tristan, she thought of the little sister playing dress up in the princess costume and asking for help with eye shadow and lipstick. Anna was Mallory's "mini-me." They were beautiful reverse images of each other, the blue-eyed blonde Mallory and the brown-eyed brunette Anna.

Andrew, child number three and the closest in age to Tristan (they were not quite six years apart), had a very different attitude. His attitude was a bit more "*que sera sera*" (whatever will be will be; if you just thought of Doris Day and started humming the song of that same name then we should definitely be friends).

The search for another therapist had begun, and the struggle was real. How would I come up with a few good choices, and how would we ever agree on one? It turns out that finding a few good choices was a pretty daunting task. Here were the criteria for the next therapist:

1. Specialize in working with teenagers.
2. Specialize in working with depression.
3. Have some experience with gender dysphoria.
4. Accepting new patients.

Looks easy, right? Criteria one and two were easy, peasy. Add in number three, and you have a bit of a challenge; not impossible, just harder to find. The deal breaker is number four. It seems like good therapists (whether they're Ph.D.s, LCSWs, LPCs, or whatever) are NEVER taking new patients.

Curious as to what's what in the world of mental health care acronyms? Here's a summary:

- Ph.D.—Doctor of Philosophy, in this case someone with a doctoral degree in social work. They work with patients/clients to deal with emotional and social problems and life changes.
- LCSW—Licensed Clinical Social Worker who work with their clients (technically they have clients, not patients, although everybody calls them patients, and no one seems to care) to find support in their social environment.
- LPC—Licensed Professional Counselors whose focus is to provide emotional and behavioral therapy support. They also have clients, not patients.

At this point I wasn't going to be picky. I didn't care if you were a Ph.D., a LCSW, an LPC, or a CEO as long as you were licensed and met the four criteria above.

The search started, as all searches have started since the 1990s, on the internet. The results pop up, and there you are, all filled with hope because there are so many to choose from! They all give you options—send an email or call and leave a message on their confidential voice mail. I left more voice mail messages than I can count. A few times I even got to speak with a friendly receptionist, whose job it was to tell me, and all of the moms like me who called for an appointment in their times of desperation, that the therapist in question was not taking new patients. Many of the voicemails were never returned, so I had my answer on those.

Of the few who did take time to call me back, one was a shining star, a glimmer of light, a beacon of hope (cliché time, again). Her name was Paula, and we talked for thirty minutes. Thirty minutes of non-billed phone time in the world of mental health professionals is an eternity. Paula seemed perfect. She specialized in teenagers, specifically those with depression, gender dysphoria, and LGBTQ issues. And she seemed to live in a place that I called reality. For the first time since this journey began, a mental health professional admitted that sometimes children and teens who begin the transgender journey don't complete it. She admitted that sometimes there are issues other than gender dysphoria, and that in our loose, progressive, modern society young people (on occasion) identify themselves as transgender when in fact there are other, deeper, underlying issues that need to be dealt with before launching into a world of gender transition. She told me that she'd worked with many teens who have truly suffered from gender dysphoria, and with a number of others who had discovered on their journey with her that they were not, in fact, transgender. Hallelujah, I had found the answer to my prayers; someone who wouldn't tell me or Tristan what we wanted to hear, but would help Tristan in her journey of self-discovery, wherever that would take her. Of course, I'm human so I'll admit that I secretly hoped that Tristan's journey would lead her back to Anna.

But, alas, Paula was not to be in our lives. You see, Paula ran two separate practices. One was as an employee of a behavioral health group which, you guessed it, had no openings for new patients. The other was a brand-new part-time counseling practice that she had just started and where she did have openings, but there was just one issue—she shared that practice with Debra, the hammer. We opted to go on a wait list and join Paula at the behavioral group, but when she finally called (after nine months of waiting) we were in too deep with Paula's runner-up to switch therapists at that point. (Plus, Tristan absolutely refused to even speak with her.)

Paula's runner-up was an LPC (license professional counselor) named James. James was, and I'm sure still is, a great guy. For some reason I envisioned a female therapist, so having a male therapist felt like a compromise, although I'm not sure why. The best part was that Tristan really seemed to like James. We had family sessions weekly and Tristan-only sessions weekly. From time to time we even had mom-and-dad-only sessions. This went on for months, and months, and months (as of this writing Tristan and James have been together for over two years). James met criteria one (teens), two (depression), and four (new patients) for sure, and he indicated to us that he had some experience with criteria three (gender dysphoria) as well.

James's demeanor was pretty neutral, and we all actually liked the fact that he called us out when we were screwing up (although truthfully, I'm not sure how much Tristan appreciated being called out). He was a go-with-the-flow kind of guy. His metaphor of choice was "planting flags," meaning when you take a position on something and hold onto it with a vengeance and refuse to look beyond the "flag" that you've planted and consider other options, you get stuck. We (Tristan, me, and Curt) spent a lot of time with James discussing how we all had a habit of "planting flags" and trying to figure out how to work through our family stalemates, or better yet how to avoid them all together.

Tristan warmed up to James pretty quickly considering the fact that she was furious when we pulled the plug on Debra not too long before. I was simply relieved that we had found a therapist that could see us ASAP. Tristan liked telling her story, so a new therapist meant a new opportunity to convince someone that she was truly a *he*.

I still wasn't convinced; this transgender revelation had seemingly come out of nowhere. We were only a few months in, and it seemed like a lifetime. By now everything in our lives revolved around Tristan being transgender. She was angry and argumentative; every situation, every conversation, every television show, every news story was a new opportunity for her to pick a fight. No matter what the topic, she managed to turn it into a transgender issue. Remember in *My Big Fat Greek Wedding* when Gus Portokalos says, "Give me a word, any word, and I show you that the root of that word is Greek"? Well, that was our life, but it was, "Give me a topic, any topic, and I'll show you how that topic is an injustice to the transgender community." I should probably expand:

- Television story about the U.S. Military–"The military is discriminating against transgender people. Now I couldn't join the military even if I wanted to."
- News story about the unemployment rate–"Transgender people are constantly discriminated against when they try to find a job."
- Any news story or mention of anything dealing with the medical profession–"You do know that there's a vote coming up in Congress to allow doctors to refuse treatment to transgender patients?"
- Announcement that other family members are joining us for dinner–"Oh, great, you know [insert name of family member here] is a total jerk who hates transgender people."

The good thing about James (good for me, at least) was that he saw Tristan's anger, and he let her know when he saw it flare up. And it was flaring up a lot—at home, at therapy, and pretty much anytime and anyplace where we were together anger was sure to follow. We were a family of hard-heads, and we planted our share of flags.

James gave us homework, too. It works both ways, this family therapy stuff, so Tristan had homework and so did Mom and Dad. As ridiculous as it may sound, our homework would be things like listening without comment to the other person, thinking before speaking, and being willing to walk away from a verbal explosion rather than participate in it. Did we really need to pay someone to tell us this stuff that intelligent adults (and intelligent teenagers who are almost adults, legally) should know instinctively? Well, we sure did. Being the hardheaded flag planters that we were, we had developed some pretty ugly patterns of interaction. So, we left every week with a homework assignment that felt a bit childish, and the next week we reported back with our results. We learned to take the good with the bad, and to try again next week if we needed to.

The bad thing about James (bad for me and for Tristan) was that James really had no experience with gender dysphoria or with the transgender community. Remember James met criteria one (teens), two (depression), and four (new patients), and he had INDICATED to us that he had some experience with criteria three (gender dysphoria) as well. I came to learn soon enough that his experience likely came more from books he had read than with clients he had worked with (remember, medical doctors have patients, therapists have clients). James often mentioned this book or that book, and how he wanted to look something up and read more about it to help Tristan. Don't get me wrong, reading and researching certainly aren't negatives. But in this case, it felt like working with Tristan was a bit of OJT (on the job training) for him, and he was diggin' it. You've gotta start somewhere, right?

If you're a therapist who's never worked with a transgender teen before and one seemingly falls out of the sky and into your office, then you certainly don't send them away. Like the rest of us, therapists have bills to pay. Landing a transgender teen with clinical depression, parental conflict, and parents who were willing to pay anything to help their child wasn't an everyday occurrence, I'm sure, in the counseling world. He seemed to really enjoy all that Tristan brought to the table for him professionally. She was a challenge he was ready and willing to accept, and even better, he was getting paid to sharpen his transgender skills. And Tristan really liked him; her whole week revolved around James's appointments.

Once again, everybody wins—or not. Because, while I'm sure that most therapists (James included) enter that profession for the noble cause of helping others who need it most, let's face reality here—it's a business. And businesses need to make money. James had a boss, he had hours to bill, he had a mortgage and a car payment. More therapy sessions mean more money. And there were sooooo many therapy sessions (and sooooo much money).

And there was sooooo little progress. I wanted progress, I prayed for progress, I looked everywhere for it, but I couldn't see it. It just wasn't happening. Every week Curt and I showed up for our family sessions with Tristan just to watch her plant the same flags and complain about the same things:

- We wouldn't call her Lucas (until she decided to be Tristan).
- We *sometimes* slipped and called her Anna instead of Tristan (ok, we had eighteen plus years of calling her Anna, so give me a break).
- We didn't believe that she'd been transgender all of her life (no, we didn't because we had seen NOTHING in her past to tell us that she identified as a male).

The weekly family sessions eventually turned to every two or three weeks, and finally I told James to put us "on call." If he had something significant come up and needed us, then I'd make an appointment and come back. After several months of sitting in a room for an hour every week listening to your teenager tell a stranger that you're basically a dirtbag, I'd had enough.

SOMEONE IS MISSING

We moved a couple of years ago, and as I was packing, I found a stack of beautifully framed photographs that had once been hanging on the wall. They were removed from the wall because someone was missing—Anna. She was missing because the photos were taken two months before she was even a twinkle in her mother's eye. In the fall of 1999 (having no idea what Y2K had in store for me) I decided that professional black and white photographs of the three kids would be a wonderful Christmas surprise for Curt. I was certain that our family was complete, so now was the perfect time to capture the little ones while they were still little ones. The photo shoot took place in a beautiful treed field with leaves falling and children smiling and playing like little angels. The photographer convinced me (I'm totally camera shy) to join in, so there we were; mama and the three angels all dressed in blue jeans and white shirts, hugging trees, throwing leaves, and smiling at the camera. All three kids kept the secret from their dad, and we surprised him on Christmas morning with photos of me and the three of them together, and of each one individually. The photo collection made a stunning collage on the wall. But, after Anna was born, it didn't seem right to have them on the wall. Someone was missing. After a few years the photos came off of the wall and went into the attic. Not long ago I hung them back on the wall. Because now even the pictures taken after Anna was born, the ones with Anna in them, have someone missing. Tristan is missing from the family photos, and Anna is missing from the family.

CHAPTER 10

THE EMT

If I could give you one thing in life, I would give you the ability to see yourself through my eyes. Only then would you realize how special you are to me.

~ Author unknown

Tristan continued to see James after Curt and I called it quits with him (as I write this, she still sees him every week). She kept a busy schedule: therapy, working part time, and school (plus visits to an endocrinologist and a psychiatrist, more on both of those coming up).

After a few months, the two part-time jobs got narrowed down to one; the pet store job was the keeper. She liked her co-workers, she got to pet dogs every day, and there were adoptable cats at the store to play with when things were slow. What more could a seventeen-year-old animal lover ask for? Oh, and I got the opportunity to see the world of dog food in a whole new light. I had no idea until that pet store job that (gasp) you NEVER feed your dog that horrible stuff they sell in the grocery store! It's practically animal abuse—I know this because Anna (she was still Anna then) told me. And right after schooling me on the evils of grocery store dog food, she shamed me into buying the primo dog food, the dog food of dog foods. Princess had somehow managed to live thirteen healthy years on that grocery store swill, but those days were gone! Do you have any idea what happens when you start your healthy thirteen-year-old pup on a new dietary regimen of the latest and greatest healthy stuff on the market, even if you ease it into their diet like a good dog mama? Well, let's just say that our vet was able to make his boat payment that month. But I'm getting off track.

In the winter *after* (after drum corps, because life at this point seems to be divided into *before drum corps* and *after drum corps*), Tristan entered an EMT (Emergency Medical Technician) program at the community college. In true Tristan fashion, she decided–moments before the application deadline–to apply for entrance into the program that being an EMT was her life's calling. And in true Tristan fashion, she got her paperwork in just in time and started working to become an EMT.

She loved the program and seemed to thrive in that environment. She took the coursework very seriously. When it came time for clinicals, she seemed to shine there as well. She was very proud of the emails that her instructor received from ambulance services and hospital emergency room personnel praising her for her compassion and diligence. Once again, we were so proud of her devotion and determination.

The only angst she had with her EMT program was that the instructor always called her Anna and referred to her as "Miss." She liked him, but that infuriated her. (Somehow, I understood, although I still couldn't bring myself to call Tristan by male pronouns.) Legally she was still Anna, showing as a female named Anna on the roster of students. He was going by what he had on paper. It didn't help, either, that she still looked like a cute girl with super short hair who dressed in boys' clothing. She had reminded him a few times that she preferred to be called Tristan, but he just couldn't (or wouldn't) get the hang of it. Finally, Tristan asked me to help her figure out how to get him to understand. We drafted an email together that seemed to help it all sink in with him, and he made a real effort going forward to address her as she wanted him to. One of life's little ironies: I couldn't do the male pronouns, but I don't want someone else to hurt my child by refusing to use them. There's really no good excuse here, just an explanation. She'd been Anna Marie to me for over eighteen years. He'd met her a few months ago.

One of the things we discussed when all of this was going on was how it might be easier if she went forward with the legal name change. Obviously as far as school was concerned, she'd show up on the class rosters as Tristan, so her instructors wouldn't know anything different. She wouldn't have to explain to her instructors and the staff at the fire/ambulance stations and hospitals that she wanted to be called a name other than the one they saw on all of her printed documents.

As far as I was concerned, I think there was a psychological component to all of this. It would be easier for me (at least I thought it would be easier) if she legally became Tristan. It would be easier for me to say *goodbye* to Anna (easier, not easy). I told myself that lots of people change their names. And Tristan sure was better than Lucas in my book. Besides, even I had wanted to change my name—twice. When I was a kid, I wanted to be Judith Marie. I thought that was the most beautiful, elegant name I'd ever heard. When I was a little older, I wanted to be Megan Elizabeth. Lots of people change their names, and even more people conjure up what their name would be if *they,* and not their parents, chose their own name. I convinced myself that a legal name change was something I could handle. But those male pronouns were a bitch. I just couldn't wrap my brain around the finality of *her* being a *him*.

Wondering how that EMT program played out? Tristan absolutely thrived in the program. She truly loved helping people, and her compassionate side shined through the darkness when she was in the "field" working with patients (ambulance ride-alongs and hospital emergency room shadowing). Her field supervisors were wonderful to her, and her colleagues in the field treated her with acceptance and respect. Her field assignments took her to neighborhoods outside of our upper-middle-class bubble, so she witnessed real life outside of the fantasyland where she grew up. She took to it like a duck to water. At age seventeen, a few weeks before her eighteenth birthday, Tristan completed the EMT certification program and passed both the state and national exams (written and practical) on the first try. Once again, we were so proud of her. (Fun fact: for the national certification to be awarded you must be eighteen or older. Tristan had to make a phone call the day of her eighteenth birthday to request that her certification be issued since she was now "legal.")

It was also about this time that Tristan began the push for male hormones. She wanted to begin a trial period of testosterone injections. A testosterone trial typically lasts three months, during which time the patient injects themselves with small but increasing amounts of testosterone to see how their body reacts and how it impacts their mental state. I'd had six months to digest all of this, and I wasn't doing a great job of it. If calling her Tristan was hard, and calling her *he* was damn near impossible, then asking me to agree to testosterone injections was like asking me to flap my arms and fly to the moon (stay with me, more to come).

NUMBER ONE FAN

Like most children I know, Anna was always a big Disney fan. Her all-time, absolute favorite Disney movie was *The Lion King*, and her favorite character was Simba. She was a *Lion King* aficionado; she had the stuffed animals, the toys, and the Simba dress-up costume. *Lion King* was her jam—until she discovered *The Phantom of the Opera*.

When Anna was around four years old, we ended up with a *Phantom* DVD. She begged to watch it, and since Curt and I had seen it ourselves and didn't see any harm we thought *what the heck, she'll likely last five minutes and demand to watch* Lion King *instead*. We could not have been more wrong; she was mesmerized. The characters and the music fascinated her, and she couldn't get enough. She was practically obsessed, and it lasted for years (actually, I'm not completely sure the obsession is over yet). The other three children liked it well enough, but not like Anna. When she was five years old there was a talent show at her school. She was determined to sing a song from *Phantom*, and she practiced nonstop. The day of the show she stood up on stage and belted out a most amazing rendition of Christine Daae's *Think of Me*. The parents sitting around me were dumbfounded. The other kids had gotten up on stage to show off a yo-yo trick or do a back flip, but not my little *prima donna, first lady of the stage* (if that line is unfamiliar to you then PLEASE grab a copy of the original *Phantom of the Opera* movie ASAP and see for yourself; it's not Broadway, but it's still pretty amazing). I'm sure the other parents thought that our whole family was a bunch of nuts.

We proved that to be true (the part about us being nuts) the following year when Anna had just turned six years old. Since she was still *Phantom*-obsessed and it clearly wasn't going away, Curt and I decided to take the whole gang plus my parents to New York City over Thanksgiving weekend to see the play on Broadway. Off we went to the Majestic Theatre, all dressed up for the show of a lifetime, and that it was. Anna wore a green velvet Christmas dress and black patent leather shoes. She was ready for action. I'd seen the play at the Majestic once before, so I was aware of their *no children under eight years old* policy. Surely, this didn't mean Anna, their number one fan. I did what a mama does when she's certain that there's no other choice—I told Anna that if anyone should dare to ask her age (they didn't), then she's eight. Just for tonight, she's eight. I knew that she'd behave like a champ, and she did. We had perfect seats, front row center mezzanine; she never took her eyes off of the stage.

After the show we discovered that my mother had buttered up one of the ushers during intermission and had found out where and when the actors would exit the building. So, we found ourselves in an alley in New York City at eleven o'clock at night waiting for the cast to show up (she should have been in bed, I know, but this was the Phantom, and Raoul, and Christine, and Carlotta). The cast was the most gracious bunch, making a huge deal over this little six-year-old who was waiting so patiently for them. They gave her hugs, signed her program, and let her pet Carlotta's doggie. I'm pretty sure that I would have gotten *Mother of the Year* if it weren't for that part about telling her to lie about her age and waiting in the alley.

CHAPTER 11

THE BUDDY

Wherever there is a human in need, there is an opportunity for kindness and to make a difference.

~ Kevin Heath

Remember James, the LPC? Well, right after Tristan started seeing him, I was talking with a friend, and that friend mentioned a wonderful therapist that she and her daughter were seeing. As it turns out, several of my friends were seeing that same therapist. Her name was Rachel. Rachel's SEO (search engine optimization) clearly wasn't as advanced as James's, or Paula's, or Debra's, or Mona's because her name never came up during my hours of internet research as I was trying to find someone who met my four basic criteria (teens, depression, gender dysphoria, new patients). Rachel, as it turns out, met all four.

Think about all of the time I could have saved if only I'd asked my friends to recommend a good therapist for my teenager! Who am I kidding, I would NEVER have asked my friends if anyone could recommend a good therapist. That's exposure, imperfection, that's for people who need help, for God's sake. And I NEVER needed help. But it's amazing what happens when you expose yourself (emotionally—don't worry, I'm not getting weird). You find out that you're not alone. Yes, I sure felt alone in the transgender teenager experience, but I sure wasn't alone in the *oh my gosh how do I even begin to help my child* experience. Turns out, lots of parents have lots of teenagers who need lots of help getting through life. There's no stigma, no embarrassment. And many of those parents are more than willing to help parents like me who are newbies at this whole therapy thing. You just have to ask.

I went to see Rachel on my own first. I might be a slow learner sometimes, but eventually I figure it out. What I'd figured out by this time was that I personally, just me, needed to meet with any/all future therapists, sit on the comfy (or not) couch, look them in the eye, and hear what they had to say. Oh, and I needed to have my say, too. No Debra would ever again worm her way into our therapy life, not on my watch. I truly *wasn't* looking for an ally (for me or for Tristan), I was looking for a savior (for me and for Tristan). I was looking for someone neutral, someone whose only agenda was to help their clients/patients get through whatever messiness was causing them angst, no matter what the outcome should happen to be. Did I still hope way deep down inside that someone, anyone, would help Tristan (God, I missed Anna so much) flip back that gender switch and be my sweet baby girl again? Oh, hell yeah. I wanted a Dr. Phil, and I was ready for a Dr. Phil beatdown; anything to get through the hell that was our lives at that point.

Since our track record with therapists wasn't exactly stellar, I had to tread lightly when I mentioned Rachel to Tristan. You see, Tristan had bonded pretty quickly with James in just a few visits, so asking her to leave him behind for yet another new beginning was ludicrous, even for me. But, there was a solution! Rachel had group therapy. I didn't need to ask Tristan to leave James. I just needed to convince her to add another therapist to the mix. After all, Tristan loved sharing her tales of transgender woe with anyone who would listen, so I was certain that I could at least get her to go and meet Rachel without too much pushback. Wrong again. Timing is everything, especially when you're tiptoeing around time bombs in your house, so I waited until the perfect time to tell Tristan about my meeting with Rachel and suggest that we both go and pay her a visit to see what this group counseling stuff was all about.

Tristan responded with the mother of all *HELL NO*s. She made it quite clear that all I wanted was to force her to switch therapists, again, and that if I liked this Rachel person then she (Tristan) wanted nothing to do with her. And since I liked her (Rachel) so much I could go and see her on my own. She had her therapist (James) so I should have my own, too. Don't ask again because this Rachel group therapy thing WAS NOT going to happen. She (Tristan) was sick and tired of my trying to find a therapist who was only on my side and just wanted to convince her that she wasn't transgender. What was I going to try next, conversion therapy?

And then, as quickly as Tornado Tristan touched ground, it dissipated. As quickly as she launched into her tirade of why she'd never, ever go and see Rachel she did a complete about-face and said that, yep, she'd go and meet her—but that was it. She'd meet her once and only once, just so that I couldn't say that she (Tristan) didn't try.

Tristan's one-time-only trial visit to Rachel took a turn that even I didn't expect. Tristan seemed sold from the beginning. I was shocked. Rachel explained in detail the dynamics of the new group that was being formed. Everyone was about Tristan's age, all between seventeen and nineteen. Each had their own unique challenges to work through, but they all had one thing in common— making and keeping friends was difficult for all of them, so that was a big focus of the group. There was no judgement allowed in the group, no negativity. Acceptance of each other was mandatory, no exceptions. Meetings were once each week, in the evening. There would ALWAYS be food, because food and teenagers just make a happy couple. And there would often be dogs, because who doesn't love dogs? What happened in the group stayed in the group. There was to be no talking about each other, no sharing of secrets, and absolutely no fraternizing with each other outside of group. Tristan was all over it; she couldn't wait to start.

Curt and I saw Rachel a few times, as well—sometimes with Tristan and sometimes without. Rachel became our common ground—something/someone that we all liked.

Other than the part about bringing your dog to group (which Tristan took full advantage of, bringing both Princess and Caly at different times), I'm pretty sure Tristan's favorite part about Rachel's group was the *Bitch Cake*. A bitch cake is a simple sheet cake, undecorated. The members of the group use icing tubes to decorate the cake with words describing all of the things that make them angry and upset, all of the things they want to bitch about. And, even though there was a strict "no fraternization among group members outside of group" rule, Tristan did make some friends in the group (that was my favorite part, because I desperately wanted her to have friendship back in her life).

Here's a quick glimpse into the life of Tristan at this point: individual therapy is weekly with James, group therapy is weekly with Rachel, EMT program is in full swing, and the part-time job is rolling right along.

And the push for a testosterone trial is stronger than ever (I told you we'd get back to that).

Rachel had gotten to know both me and Tristan pretty well, and she knew that both Curt and I struggled with the thought of Tristan starting hormone treatments. We knew it was inevitable, but we just couldn't bear the thought of making that decision for our seventeen-year-old. Tristan continually planted her *I want to start testosterone treatments* flag while we planted our *then do it when you're eighteen because we're not signing for it* flag. Poor Rachel got to hear this from both sides, over and over. Rachel (like a good therapist) had not taken a stance one way or the other. Tristan was only a few months away from turning eighteen by this point, so we were really just biding our time until the decision wasn't ours to make. And then one day Rachel called me on the phone. She had just attended a professional convention and one of the speakers was the director of a non-profit organization for teenagers in the LGBTQ community. Let's call it We Support You (WSU). The WSU Director spoke about testosterone trials for transgender teenagers, and he was not a fan. Quite the opposite, he was a strong advocate of trans-gender teens waiting until age eighteen to begin testosterone treat-ment. Rachel offered to arrange for all of us (me, Curt, Tristan, Rachel) to meet with a counselor from WSU in hopes of bringing us all some peace. Rachel felt certain that the counselor would support the opinion of the director, so maybe we'd all benefit from hearing why the director of WSU had taken the stance of *wait until you're eighteen to start testosterone.*

Another one of life's little ironies: Tristan (before she was Tris-tan, when she was still Anna/Lucas) had months earlier hounded me (incessantly, as is her style) to visit WSU for the education and support that I clearly needed. She thought it would be a great way for me to learn more about the transgender community and that their parent support groups would help me a great deal. I told her the truth: I just wasn't ready for that. I was completely shell-shocked by all of this, and emotionally I was hanging on by a thread. She wasn't asking me to go and learn how to swing dance (I'd failed miserably at that years ago, anyway), she was asking me to go and learn how to watch my daughter become my son. Even the thought of that was more than I could handle. But wait, there's more! Although I wasn't ready/willing to jump in and find my new BFFs at WSU, I suggested that Tristan (Anna/Lucas) go and visit to get both the support and friendship that she so desperately needed (since education on the topic was one thing she did not need; she knew more than enough about the transgender community). Her response: the same HELL NO of the Rachel HELL NO, but this time it was firm, and she was not changing her mind. She had no interest in WSU, and nothing in common with the people who went there. Tristan's opinion: the members had formed more of a political extremist group than an emotional support group and there was nothing for her to gain by visiting their groups. Well, okay then.

Rachel got us an appointment to meet with Carolyn, a counselor at WSU, for what we thought/hoped would be some clarity and affirmation about the benefits of waiting until age eighteen to start hormone therapy. I knew by now that this hormone thing was going to happen, so I had no expectation that Carolyn or anyone else would dissuade Tristan (Anna) from going through with it. All I hoped for at that point was some peace in our house for the next few months, something to end this testosterone argument for the time being. I'll speak the unspoken here, too: I also hoped that those few months might give Tristan (Anna) time to rethink this whole thing. Knowing that testosterone treatments are on the horizon was one thing, but it was another thing entirely to allow it to happen. How could I sign paperwork to let my seventeen-year-old start testosterone treatments? A seventeen-year-old is . . . a seventeen-year-old. They change their minds hourly. I was seventeen once, I remember. I couldn't bear the thought that one day she might come back to me and say, "Why? Why did you let me do that? I was seventeen. It was your job to make the big grownup decisions, and you screwed up."

Carolyn was young; she looked barely older than seventeen herself. She was friendly, compassionate, and understanding. And she was a complete advocate of testosterone treatments for the eighteen-and-under crowd. I was blown away. What did I want? I wanted someone to tell us all that Tristan was too young to shoot herself up with male hormones. What did I expect (based on my talk with Rachel, which was based on her talk with the director)? I expected someone who was neutral on the topic. What did I get? I got an introduction to teen suicide rates among gender dysphoric individuals and a mini-version of the "sex talk" which included a multicolored cartoon animal (let's call it an elephant because I honestly don't remember due to my dumbfounded state of being at the time). How did we end up with a multicolored cartoon elephant? Carolyn was explaining the difference between gender identity and sexual orientation (in a nutshell: a transgender male [AFAB, assigned female at birth] may be attracted to females or may be attracted to males; same goes for a transgender female).

I left WSU even more confused than I was when I went in.

PEOPLE SURPRISE YOU

Sometimes younger generations greatly misjudge older generations, which I know from first-hand experience. When it was time to tell the grandparents that Anna was now Tristan, and Tristan intended to live as a male, I was pretty sure that they'd struggle with the whole concept. How could they not? I was struggling, Curt was struggling, and even our other kids were struggling. I dreaded telling them, but clearly, they had to be told sooner rather than later. Now we had to try and explain the whole transgender concept to my parents and Curt's dad (Curt's mom had passed away several years before). How do you explain something that you absolutely can't understand yourself?

I have no idea what reaction I expected from the grandparents, but the reaction I got pretty much blew me away. Sure, they were confused. But they were also kind and accepting. They all handled the news much better than I had when I was told. They all seemed to take the name change in stride, and one of them immediately began using male pronouns as if *she* had been a *he* since day one. None of them seemed uncomfortable with Tristan's new identity, and if they had any negative feelings or thoughts they did a great job of keeping them to themselves. They clearly love and support their grandchild, no matter what, and I hope that Tristan realizes what a blessing that is.

CHAPTER 12

THE SHRINK

Even the darkest night will end, and the sun will rise.

~ Victor Hugo, *Les Miserables*

I don't remember how we found Dr. Davidson, but I know why we found her. Tristan, back when she was Anna, needed to see a medical doctor who could prescribe medication to treat her depression. In the very early days of the depression diagnosis, Mona had worked with Tristan's PCP (primary care physician) to prescribe some mild antidepressants. Mona did the counseling, and Dr. Fay, the PCP, wrote the prescriptions. The two of them shared information as they looked for a balance of therapy and meds that would help. Somewhere along the line (I believe it was after Mona and before James), we came to the conclusion that it would be easier to find a therapist who was a medical doctor. That would be a psychiatrist, or so you would think.

Psychiatrists are medical doctors who are able to prescribe medications, which they do in conjunction with providing psychotherapy, though medical and pharmacological interventions are often their focus. (VeryWellMind.com)

When Tristan (she was going by Lucas now) started seeing Dr. Davidson I naïvely assumed that Dr. Davidson (being a psychiatrist) would provide some level of therapy along with writing prescriptions. But, alas, that was not to be. I accompanied Tristan on the first few visits, and we were in and out in a flash. The doc spoke with Tristan for a few moments, didn't give me the time of day, and was out of the door quicker than you can say, "Let's up your dosage." Clearly, I was confused when I assumed that Dr. Davidson would do something other than ask Tristan a few questions and then write a prescription (you know what happens when you assume? I learned the answer from Felix Unger on *The Odd Couple* when I was about seven—when you assume you make an Ass of U and Me). Yep, I felt like an ass. I had just sat there and said/did nothing while Dr. Flash did her thing. And her thing involved a pen and a prescription pad, nothing more. No therapy, no counseling, no conversation beyond the few questions she asked Anna about her current medication and how it was or wasn't helping.

The first time this happened I let it go. But the next time I was ready. I had my list of questions, and I was determined to get some answers. I asked my questions, and all of the answers were the same: go and ask your therapist. Dr. Davidson had no intention of providing any type of counseling services. She was writing prescriptions and that was it. The more questions I asked, the more dismissive she became. She came into the room, spoke briefly with Anna/Lucas, made it very clear that she had no interest in speaking with me AT ALL, wrote the latest prescription and out of the door she went. She was cold, rigid, and indifferent; I absolutely despised her. And, I got the impression that the feeling was mutual. She seemed irritated every time I opened my mouth to speak, as if my questions and concerns were of no consequence to her. I once even followed her out of the exam room (the audacity; I had the nerve to want to ask questions about my daughter's mental health treatment) to try and ask a question since she brushed me off when I tried to ask the question in the room. Her reaction to that? She ignored me as I called her name, not five feet behind her, and went into another room and shut the door. I get it, schedules to keep and all of that, but come on! I then walked over to the check-out desk and explained that I had a question for the doctor and would like to speak with her. The answer? Write down your name and number on this little piece of paper and we'll have her call you. That was my last visit to Dr. Davidson, although Tristan continued to see her and still does. FYI, she never called me.

There are good doctors and bad ones, doctors who want to help and doctors who just want to make their Porsche payments. We definitely helped Dr. Flash with the latter.

THE THIRD TIME

One day, when Anna was barely four years old, she and I were at the mall—alone. This was quite the rarity since a mama of four doesn't often get solo time with any of the bunch. Out of the blue she asked if she could get her ears pierced. We called Curt to get his input; I explained to her that this was a big deal and that both parents should agree before we started putting holes in her body. With both parents' blessing, she marched down to the store, jumped up on the stool, and sat there like a champ. But there was a problem. The store only had one piercing technician on duty, which meant each ear would be pierced one at a time rather than their preferred *one tech on each ear and one two three go* both holes get done at the same time. Anna insisted that she was having them pierced right then and there, no matter what. Until the first ear was pierced. She refused to let the tech pierce number two, so earring number one (gold post and pink stone) was removed and we went home.

A few weeks later she was ready again, this time with two technicians. *One two three go* and she had an adorable gold teddy bear in each ear. Until a few days later when we all went to see a movie. Anna decided that she wanted to see the gold teddy bears, so out they came. By the time I realized that she had removed the earrings, one of the teddy bears had been lost and the holes in her ears had closed up. When the ear-piercing tech tells you to keep the earrings in for six weeks and NEVER take them out during that time, they mean business.

The third time was the charm. A few months after the teddy bear incident, Anna and Curt were alone at the mall. You guessed it, she wanted to get her ears pierced again. By now Anna's ear piercing was old news, so they clearly didn't need to call and check in with mama. Off they went to the store, and they came home to surprise me with Anna sporting her new gold and pink studs. This time the technician put locking backs on the earrings, and we gave Anna a mirror so she could keep watch over them.

Tristan, even when she was a little girl named Anna, has never been one to take "no" for an answer. Heck, she won't even take "later" for an answer. She's strong willed and determined, and she WILL eventually get what she wants. She definitely has an iron will. I love that about her, except when I don't love it; and then I absolutely despise it. When she makes up her mind there's absolutely no stopping her. Her determination keeps me on my toes (and sometimes makes me question my decisions). Her spirit is both exhilarating and exhausting at the same time. One thing is certain: when she sets her mind to something, she is a force to be reckoned with. If she wants something, she's going to do what it takes to make it happen. Whatever path she follows in life, I have a feeling she'll be just fine.

CHAPTER 13

THE PUSHER

God grant me the serenity to accept the things I cannot change,
courage to change the things I can, and wisdom
to know the difference.

~Reinhold Niebuhr

By now Tristan had so many appointments with so many different health care professionals (weekly individual therapy with James, weekly group therapy with Rachel, appointments every couple of months with Dr. Flash, the shrink) that she had her own color code in my Google calendar (her color was yellow). It was time to add another to our list of medical professionals; now we had an endocrinologist in the mix.

After our escapade at WSU, Tristan was more insistent than ever on starting hormone therapy. Who wouldn't be, with that multicolored cartoon elephant, and all? It was the same battle every day; she wanted to start taking testosterone, and I wanted her to wait a few months until her birthday (we were about three months away from the big eighteenth at that time).

Tristan and I met with Dr. Smith, an endocrinologist who happened to work in the same practice as Dr. Davidson (I'll never learn), to discuss how all of this would work. Just to discuss it, that was it. Dr. Smith was not nearly as cold as Dr. Davidson (the psychiatrist), but she clearly had one agenda only, and that was to get the testosterone party started.

One conversation that I'd had with Tristan (a few times) regarding her gender dysphoria was haunting me. I'd asked her if she felt 100% certain that this (living as a male) was her true path in life. Seventeen-year-olds have been known to change their direction from time to time, and not all people (young or old) who start down the path of gender transition end up following it to the end. Some of them realize, as they take their path, that their assigned gender at birth is truly the one that they identify with. This isn't a common occurrence, but it isn't unheard of either. Gender dysphoria can be (at times) symptomatic of something else. So, I asked her if she was 100% certain of her male identity. And her answer was this: no one can ever be 100% certain of anything.

Do you buy that? Because I don't. There are things that I believe with 100% certainty. I believe that there is a God. I believe that having faith in your life can help you make it through the darkest times, and that a life without faith will always be a life of struggle. I believe that love is the most powerful emotion that any of us can ever experience, and when you have it in your life, you'd better not let it go. I believe that for every person in this world there is another person out there who is destined to be theirs, and I thank God every day that I found mine. I believe that my children are a blessing, all four of them, and that, for some reason I'll never know, God gave them to me because he thought I could handle it. No one will ever convince me that you cannot be 100% certain of anything.

How do you decide to change your gender (if that's really even possible, given DNA and all of that) while at the same time admit that you're not 100% certain of anything in your life?

The good thing about Dr. Smith was that she was willing to listen to my questions, and she'd even answer them. I think that my most interesting question to her was this: what is the requirement, other than parental agreement, for an underage child to undergo testosterone treatment? (How long did she, the endocrinologist, need to see the patient before agreeing that this was the right course of treatment? How much therapy was required beforehand? You know, mom-type questions.) And the answer was this: there was no minimum amount of time, no minimum number of visits for the endocrinologist to get to know the patient before beginning treatment. If we'd been willing, then the treatments could have started the first time we walked through the door. Oh, and therapy beforehand? The only requirement was that a therapist, ANY therapist, write a letter to the endocrinologist giving the thumbs-up for the testosterone to start. Whether that therapist had seen the client/patient one time or one hundred times, it mattered not. And guess what Dr. Smith had in her hot little patient file? A letter from Dr. Davidson with her testosterone seal of approval. This lack of due diligence on their part offered me no comfort at all. I was scared to death of the long-term effects of testosterone, so Dr. Smith suggested a three-month trial. She explained that three months of testosterone would have minimal long-term effects (voice might be a little deeper, more acne, maybe some facial hair—those didn't sound minimal to me). First, there would be a full panel of bloodwork to rule out anything else that might be lurking in the physiological background. Dr. Smith admitted that there was the slight possibility of some type of imbalance that could be causing Tristan's gender dysphoria and depression (an example would be abnormally low estrogen levels; this would show up in the bloodwork if it did indeed exist).

The bloodwork was done, and the follow-up appointment was scheduled to discuss the results. Did I desperately hope (secretly, I never shared this with Tristan) that the bloodwork would come back and: *Eureka! The problem was low estrogen (or something equally benign) all along! Give her a shot or two and I'd have my Anna back!* I not only hoped it, I prayed it, too. But, since hopes and dreams so often elude us and prayers sometimes go unanswered, this was not even close to what happened next. During the two weeks that we were waiting for the results of the bloodwork to come back, Tristan was on a mission to make sure that this whole testosterone thing didn't die with the bloodwork. She pounded me every day, insisting that I was just using this bloodwork as a delay tactic, that I never intended to even consider a testosterone trial in the first place. The more she pounded, the more I resisted. Injecting testosterone into a female body is a scary thing, and I was absolutely terrified. Do you know what the risks and long-term physical impact of testosterone therapy on the female body are? Well, here they are, straight from the Mayo Clinic:

Risks:

- Producing too many red blood cells (polycythemia).
- Weight gain.
- Acne.
- Developing male-pattern baldness.
- Sleep apnea.
- Elevated liver function tests.
- An abnormal amount of lipids in the blood (dyslipidemia), with a higher risk in those who have polycystic ovary syndrome.
- Worsening of an underlying manic or psychotic condition.
- High blood pressure (hypertension), type 2 diabetes, and cardiovascular disease, when risk factors are present.
- The risk of permanent infertility increases with long-term use of hormones, especially when hormone therapy is initiated before puberty.

Physical Impact:

- Oily skin and acne. This will begin one to six months after treatment. The maximum effect will occur within one to two years.
- Cessation of your period. This will occur within two to six months of treatment.
- Voice deepens. This will begin three to twelve months after treatment. The maximum effect will occur within one to two years.
- Facial and body hair growth. This will begin three to six months after treatment. The maximum effect will occur within three to five years.
- Body fat redistribution. This will begin within three to six months. The maximum effect will occur within two to five years.
- Clitoral enlargement and vaginal atrophy. This will begin three to six months after treatment. The maximum effect will occur within one to two years.
- Increased muscle mass and strength. This will begin within six to twelve months after treatment. The maximum effect will occur within two to five years.
- Scalp hair loss. This will occur within twelve months of treatment.

Finally, our two weeks were up. It was D-Day, time to go back to Dr. Smith and learn Tristan's fate. She had been more belligerent than ever, convinced that I'd never agree to the testosterone trial. There's an interesting detail here. According to the medical doctors that we consulted, if an underage child is seeking testosterone treatment and is in the custody of both parents, then both parents were required to sign off in order for the child to begin the treatments. It actually brought me some comfort knowing that even if I agreed to it, there was no way in hell that Curt would agree. Theoretically, I was his scapegoat and he was mine. Testosterone would just have to wait a few months.

But then, I was sitting in Dr. Smith's office, waiting for her to come in and give us the results of the bloodwork, listening to Tristan rant about the unfairness of it all, how intolerant and bigoted I was, how I didn't love her and only wanted to control her —and then this "thing" happened. I'd been pounded for two weeks, nonstop, every waking moment in our household had been consumed with testosterone-speak. Tristan was consumed, she was obsessed, it was all she thought about, all she talked about, all she pounded about. And Dr. Smith walked into the room, began her testosterone-speak as if this whole thing was a done deal while Tristan continued to rant to the good doctor about the horrible, uncaring person that I was. And I lost it. At that moment I had the closest thing I've ever had to an out-of-body experience. And, oh boy, was it ugly.

I just couldn't take it. I was overwhelmed. I wanted to scream, I wanted to run, I just wanted out. I stood up, I opened my mouth, and the words that came out surprise me even now. I went into a raging fit. I screamed, I cursed, I told them both in no uncertain terms what I thought of all of them and of this whole situation. I screamed at Tristan for the nasty, vile behavior that I was the target of on a daily basis. I screamed and cursed Dr. Smith for being so casually willing to put Tristan through these permanent life changes and throw caution to the wind with blatant disregard for the potential long-term negative consequences. I cursed Dr. Davidson in her absences (but no worries, because the walls were old and paper-thin, and Dr. Davidson just happened to be seeing a patient in the next room so it was just like she was there for the whole thing!) for her coldness, her refusal to even have a conversation with me, for seeing my child as a statistic and not as a smart, beautiful being who was screaming out for help as she screamed at the world around her.

I have never before in my entire life acted like that, and I hope that I never do it again. But I did it, and I own it. As I was walking out the door, both Tristan and Dr. Smith looking at me as if I had three heads, Dr. Smith very politely asked me if I'd like to know the results of Tristan's bloodwork. I composed myself, and told her yes, but only if she could provide it in fifteen seconds or less, because that was exactly how long she had before I walked out the door. She's quite efficient; she took less than ten seconds to tell me that everything was exactly normal. At that point I threw my shoulders back, firmed up my shaky jelly-legs, and walked out of the building. I got in my car, called Curt, and burst into tears. I was hysterical. This is a hard thing to admit for a tough cookie like me. I pride myself on being able to handle anything life throws at me without breaking a sweat. Curt and I had been married for over thirty years by then, and he'd never seen me melt down like this. He told me to stay put because he was coming to get me. But I just needed to get out of that parking lot, away from that building and all of the coldness and heartlessness that was inside of it, as quickly as I could, so I put on my big-girl pants and drove myself home. I spent the rest of the day at home, alone, wondering how life could change so quickly in such a short period of time.

That day just happened to be a triple play for Tristan: she saw Dr. Smith, then James, then group with Rachel, all back-to-back. That was a good thing, a blessing really, because I don't think either one of us could face the other that afternoon. I'm pretty sure she thought that I'd gone stark raving mad. Not that she said this to me with her words, but instead because of what happened later that day. Shortly after her appointment with James I got a phone call—from James. He just wanted to "check-in" and see how things were going. Then, shortly after her group session with Rachel I got a phone call—from Rachel. She, too, just wanted to "check-in" and see how things were going. It really was sweet of both of them to check on me after my meltdown, but by that time I had calmed down and accepted my behavior for what it was—a mama who just flat out lost her shit. I had forgiven myself by then, and it actually felt good to let it out. I assured them both that I had not fallen off of the deep end, that I was sure whatever Tristan had told them had happened was 100% true, and that I owned my behavior, I would not apologize for it, and that there was nothing I said that I wished to take back. I think they were really just making sure that I wasn't homicidal.

THE PINK DRESS

When the children were youngish (from five years old to fifteen) Curt and I went to a charity auction, and we bought a portrait package from a local photographer. This particular package included a photograph that would then be expertly painted in oils by an artist on his staff. We neglected to read the fine print, and our package included an eight- by ten-inch photo, which would have meant that each child's head would have been approximately the size of a dime. This was pointed out to me when I called to schedule the photo shoot. Since I had envisioned a grand oil painting of my four beautiful children displayed proudly above the fireplace, this wouldn't do at all. In came the upsell. After shelling out a few more thousand dollars (yes, thousand) for the appropriately-sized portrait, we were good to go.

We spent a lot of time (we being me) ensuring that all four kids were color coordinated and had the appropriate haircuts and shoes for the photo shoot. It was a beautiful early fall day, and the photos were to be set in a patch of emerald-green grass with a few newly fallen leaves on the ground to add just the right touch of gold and orange. The color coordination of the outfits centered around five-year-old Anna, since: 1) she was the only one who gave a rip about what anyone wore for the photo, and 2) she had a dress with coordinating shoes that was her absolute favorite outfit, and that was the only outfit that she was willing to wear. Fifteen-year-old Christopher looked very grown-up in a gold sweater borrowed from Curt and a bowl-ish haircut that was quite in style at the time. Mallory, age thirteen, found a pink mock turtleneck and a silver necklace with a pink stone in my closet to go with her khaki pants; her shiny blonde hair looked lovely with the other colors in the background. Eleven-year-old Andrew chose a burgundy collared shirt which he had in his own closet; he looked very dapper with his round eyeglasses and cherub smile. And last, but not least, was Anna in her favorite outfit. She wore a pale pink velvet jumper-style dress with a white blouse underneath, a dainty silver necklace, white tights, and glittery pink shoes. She was the picture-perfect little sister.

After months of waiting it was time to pick up the painting with its ornate gold frame and take it home to hang in its place of honor. It was as beautiful as I had hoped; my four beautiful children captured in oil on canvas for eternity. After a few years the painting was replaced with a television over the fireplace. The painting just moved then to an even more prominent place in the entrance hall, guaranteeing that everyone who walked through the front door would see that first.

Now the painting hangs in the hallway upstairs just outside of our bedroom door. I see it every day, so many times every day. But, it's different now; at least one part of it is different. The little girl in the pink dress with the tremendous smile is still smiling back at me; she looks like Anna but she's not Anna. I'm not sure who she is because she's not Tristan either; Tristan isn't a girl, yet this child wearing pink sparkly shoes is definitely not a little boy. I'm not sure how much longer I can stand to look at that painting every day.

CHAPTER 14

THE HORMONES

Just because someone carries it well
Does not mean it isn't heavy.

~ Author unknown

My little meltdown in Dr. Smith's office was never brought up except by James and Rachel that one time when they called to do my safety check. Tristan never mentioned it, and I sure wasn't going to bring that up again. Dr. Smith never mentioned it, nor did Dr. Davidson, because I never laid eyes on either one of them again. Dr. Smith eventually left the practice (she moved away) and Dr. Davidson sent paperwork home to be signed allowing Tristan to be seen without a parent or guardian present. But just because we didn't talk about "the thing" doesn't mean that life at home got any better. It had been hell before the bloodwork episode, and now it was a new kind of hell. Tristan was relentless by this point. We were nine months post the transgender announcement, she was a few months away from turning eighteen, and IT NEVER STOPPED.

"IT" was the constant agonizing, pushing, pounding, demanding that we allow her to begin a three-month testosterone trial. The only real communication between Tristan, Curt, and me revolved around testosterone.

One day I just broke. The paperwork had been there for weeks, waiting for my signature (and Curt's, too—remember, both parents had to sign). I just couldn't take it anymore. And, although I believed with all of my heart that testosterone wasn't going to be the magic bullet that made Tristan happy, I couldn't see anything else in her life that made her happy, either. I was tired. Tired of the anger. Tired of the confusion. Tired of being tired. So, one day after a particularly nasty barrage from my youngest, I'd just had enough. I picked up the paperwork, grabbed a red pen (red is the color of anger, right?), signed on the dotted line, and handed it to her. No, actually I think I threw it at her like a five-year-old—although I think that most five-year-olds have better manners than that.

With one parental signature in hand, Tristan only needed Dad to sign. That part was easier than I thought it would be. I simply told Curt that I had given up, that I couldn't take it anymore, and that if he didn't sign then I would likely have a nervous breakdown, need to be institutionalized, and then he would be left to deal with this all on his own. Sadly, every word of that was true. I literally could not go on like this any longer. Curt, caught between a *Scylla and Charybdis* (you know, a rock and a hard place, mentioned in the Police song from the '80s), realized that he and I needed to stay on the same team with this so he signed, too. FYI, he used a pen with blue ink like a grown-up.

Of course, my signature came with strings attached. I may have signed the paperwork, but using red ink to convey my disapproval just wasn't going to cut it for me. I may have signed for the testosterone trial, but in no way did I approve of it. I had simply given up. I was a control freak who had lost control. If Tristan was going through with this then I certainly wasn't going to foot the bill. The only thing I had control of was the purse strings at this point. If she wanted it bad enough then she'd need to pay for it herself. Unbeknown to me at the time, testosterone injections are relatively inexpensive. Tristan made more than enough at her part-time job to cover it.

Tristan, triumphant in the battle of the hormones, was understandably anxious to get this process underway as quickly as she could. Here's how that whole thing works. An endocrinologist is the medical doctor who administers and supervises the testosterone trial. The first time a patient gets the testosterone shot someone is required to accompany them to the office, wait in the waiting room while the shot is administered, then wait with the patient for a short period of time to be sure that there are no adverse side effects. The patient leaves with a prescription for the vials of testosterone solution that they will then inject themselves in the comfort of their own home over the course of the next few weeks and months. The early doses are low and increase as the weeks go on. The frequency of the injections is typically every couple of weeks for the three-month trial period. The purpose of the three-month trial is to see how the patient reacts mentally as well as physically to the treatment (acne, facial hair growth, headache, increased blood pressure, etc.). If the trial period goes well and the negative side effects are minimal (or hopefully nonexistent) AND if the patient's mental/emotional state is improved, then the patient and the endocrinologist will decide if long-term testosterone treatment is called for.

By now Tristan was very independent when it came to handling all of these doctors and therapists. The bloodwork had already been done and the results were all fine, so when it was time to schedule the testosterone trial there was really only one detail to figure out—who would accompany Tristan the first time? Dr. Smith hadn't moved away yet and was still in the picture, so she was the one who would get the party started. I assumed (remember what happens when you assume) that I'd be the wingman who'd accompany Tristan to the first testosterone visit. I knew that I'd need to swallow my pride after my last visit with Dr. Smith, but I was ready (not anxious, but willing) to do that. Boy, did I miss the mark on that one. When I told Tristan that I would go with her for the initial treatment (silly me, I thought that I was simply stating the obvious), she responded with a definitive "HELL NO." I was a little confused, thinking maybe she'd rather have Curt go with her. Wrong again. She didn't want either one of us to go. She wanted James (the therapist with all of the flags) to go with her. Her explanation: she wanted someone there with her who was supportive and happy for her because this was to be the happiest day of her life. She knew that we didn't really want her to do this, so she didn't want us there to rain on her parade. Fair enough. I didn't want her to do this testosterone trial, and I certainly couldn't fake a happy dance while it was happening.

I may sound hypocritical to say that I felt rejected when Tristan chose James over me, but I sure did. You really can't have it both ways, can you? But I wanted it both ways. I didn't want her to start the testosterone trial, but I didn't want her to do it without me being there, either. It felt like a slap in the face. I was pretty sure that Tristan wasn't planning to nominate me for "Mother of the Year," but for God's sake I was still her mother. Kids need their mother when they get shots, don't they?

LIFE GOES ON

I was listening to a morning radio show not long ago. It was December, the year 2019 was coming to a close, and we were about to usher in a new decade. The hosts were discussing past decades and what each decade represented from a *cultural* perspective. They were trying to figure out what the 2010s represented as we left that decade behind. For the sake of space, I'll go back just few:

- 1960s: Hippies, the Vietnam War, protests
- 1970s: Disco, Roe vs. Wade, Watergate
- 1980s: Twenty-four-hour news channels, the AIDS epidemic, the fall of the Berlin Wall
- 1990s: Technology/internet, bombings, mass shootings
- 2000s: The War on Terror, Facebook/Twitter/Google, same-sex marriage

Interesting summary, right? So, what was the decade from 2010 to 2019 *the decade of*? Was it *the me decade*? The *dare to be different decade*? The *standout decade*? The *anything goes decade?* The *who gives a shit what other people think decade*? How's this for a summary:

- 2010s: iPad, meat dresses (remember Lady Gaga?), ice bucket challenges, British royal weddings, the world not ending on 12/21/12 as the Mayan calendar predicted, false missile warnings, #metoo, Pokémon Go (sorry, I just couldn't narrow the list any more than this)

I'm not sure what you think, but I think maybe we're all screwed.

CHAPTER 15

THE APARTMENT

In three words I can sum up everything I've learned about life:
it goes on.

~ Robert Frost

The three-month testosterone trial ended just as Tristan celebrated her one-year anniversary of transgender declaration. We'd now been through four seasons of transition with Tristan. She had her EMT certification and a decent job with decent hours at the pet store. Now she was searching for an apartment. The thought of her moving out at barely eighteen was a little weird, even though I'd had three others move out at eighteen. I think the difference was that the other three had moved into college housing, which is the natural next step for a lot of eighteen-year-olds. They get to test the waters of freedom away from Mom and Dad, but not too far away from Mom and Dad. Home is still home, and college is just college; it feels temporary. Tristan's move seemed more permanent. She wasn't going off to college, she was leaving home. She wasn't testing the waters; she was building her own ark.

Life at home wasn't fun, for Tristan or for me. The apartment was actually a good thing; we'd both get the separation we so desperately needed. The tension at home was never-ending. Everything, every conversation, revolved around something transgender related; that part had only intensified. Tristan decided to continue with the testosterone treatments, and since she had just turned eighteen it was all up to her. I was seeing no progress with the therapists; she was seeing James for weekly individual sessions and Rachel for weekly group sessions. By the time she moved out, Tristan was barely speaking to us. Her reasoning? He/him/his. Curt and I still couldn't stomach the male pronouns. We called her Tristan. After all, that was her legal name at this point. But when I looked at the child I had raised as Anna Marie, the he/him/his just wouldn't come out of my mouth. I just avoided pronouns. And, from time to time, I opened my mouth to speak to her and "Anna" came out; or something like "AnnnnnTRISTAN" because my brain just hadn't fully adjusted yet.

Tristan found an apartment that I felt good about. Two of our other kids had actually lived there during their college years so I knew it well. Safety was on my mind, but parents always worry about their kids' safety and this was no different. What I worried most about was loneliness—Tristan's loneliness. She was adamant that she would NOT have a roommate, that she wanted a small one-bedroom place. She was also adamant that she could afford it; we had agreed to a monthly allowance and the rest was up to her. Obviously, the allowance would go a lot further with a roommate, but she wasn't budging on that one. I worried about her isolating herself from the world. She didn't have close friends, only the people she worked with and the members of her weekly therapy group. Isolation was my biggest fear for her. Everybody needs interaction, even extreme introverts like Tristan (and me). She couldn't even take Caly with her; this was a no-dog apartment building. Besides, dogs need to be around people, they need walks, they need to go out to potty, and they can't stay alone in an apartment all day. Tristan's schedule was definitely not dog friendly. So Caly, the fluffy white fixer-of-everything, stayed with me and Curt. I will admit, keeping this little ball of joy was in no way a sacrifice for me.

One of the perks of working at the pet store was that Tristan got her daily kitten fix. The store always had cages of kitties waiting for adoption, and Tristan decided that this new apartment, with its kitten-friendly policy, needed a kitten to make it complete. This is how Freyja came to be Tristan's feline companion. Freyja, with her pale orange fur and golden eyes, her funny, in-your-face personality, and her obnoxious screaming meow, was Tristan's perfect roommate.

More changes were on the horizon. A few months after moving into the apartment Tristan gave up her job at the pet store to become a barista at Starbucks. It was a very forward-thinking move, and Tristan was planning for the future. You see, Starbucks is famous for much more than making a killer pumpkin spice latte in October. Starbucks is one of the most LGBTQ-friendly employers that you can find. And they offer a great benefits package, even if you're not full time. Their health insurance plan is top-notch. Tristan realized that she needed to have the pieces to the puzzle lined up so that she could fully gender transition when the time came, and great health insurance was the first piece to that.

I was surprised that she didn't go to work as an EMT, but that wasn't my decision to make. Since Tristan had already earned her EMT certification, she decided to take the next step and become a paramedic. She was taking some classes toward that certification while she worked at Starbucks. This was also about the time that Tristan basically quit speaking to me. She communicated when she needed something, but other than that she went on radio silence. I reached out to both James and Rachel, but now she was eighteen. That meant that they wouldn't/couldn't give me the time of day. I hit the wall. My train of thought was this: Tristan had now been in therapy for fifteen months (in addition to the eighteen months with Mona), fifteen months that I hoped would have helped her in some way deal with all of this anger and frustration that seemed to consume her. But it wasn't helping. Her attitude had gone from bad to worse. Obviously, I preferred no communication to the screaming belligerence that we'd had before, but the reality was that neither was an acceptable option. I decided to do the only thing I could think of—pull those purse strings a little tighter. I informed Tristan, Rachel, and James that Tristan had thirty days to figure out a new payment plan. If Tristan couldn't even speak to me then the therapy well was going dry. All of this therapy was being paid for out of pocket, and it was quite the monthly bill. After fifteen months and thousands upon thousands of dollars I expected more. What happened next was interesting.

James went right to work to try and figure out a payment plan that Tristan could afford. Being part of a large practice, they had dealt with this before. A therapist with free hours on the calendar is a therapist who is missing billable hours, and partial payment is better than no payment at all. They came up with a plan for Tristan that cut the hourly rate by about seventy percent—yes, seventy. Once again, everybody wins. Tristan keeps her therapist, I'm no longer paying for negative results, and James gets to keep the weekly slot full. Although he wasn't making nearly as much for that hour, he wasn't losing money either. And while Tristan could afford James's new price, she wasn't too keen on paying the bill herself. But she liked James and he had become part of her weekly routine. She wasn't giving that up, and if she had to pay for it herself then so be it. I had hoped for a different outcome. My hope was that Tristan and James would part ways, and that maybe then we'd find a therapist who would truly be of some help. I saw James as another weekly paid playdate, just as Mona had become. I didn't think James was doing any harm, but he certainly wasn't doing any good.

The result with Rachel was a little different. Her practice was independent, she was in it alone, so all of the decisions were hers. She told Tristan that, as much as she'd like to allow her to come to group, the group rate was the group rate and it wasn't being reduced just because Tristan was now responsible for the bill. I was a little surprised, but I totally respect Rachel's right to make her own decisions about how she runs her business. Tristan left the group. Surprisingly, Tristan seemed to take it all in stride. She wasn't exactly sharing her thoughts and feelings with me at that point, but when she told me about it she certainly wasn't upset to stop seeing Rachel.

THE PERFECT NAME

When I was pregnant, all four times, I was asked the same questions a zillion times: "Do you know if you're having a boy or a girl? What are you going to name him/her?" Those are the questions that everyone asks every pregnant woman they know, right? Logical questions since I'm pretty sure that every pregnant woman on earth wonders whether she's having a boy or a girl and at some point comes up with a list of potential names.

Baby names are special, aren't they? Whether the little fella is the fourth in line named after dad and grandpa and great grandpa, or whether the little angel is given one of those names that make people say, "What in the hell were her parents thinking when they named her THAT?" baby names are important to their parents. No one ever names a baby and then says, "We didn't really like that name, but we were tired of trying to decide so we just opened the baby name book and pointed to one." Parents typically agonize over baby names.

Other than pronouns, I think name changes are the hardest adjustment for parents of transgender children. Hard as it is, I actually encouraged Anna to go through with the legal name change to Tristan. I knew that she needed to make it legal for so many practical reasons, but I thought that, emotionally, it would be easier for me to accept the new name if it were official. Sound silly? It probably is silly, but in my mind, it made things easier for me. It became easier to call her Tristan when she was actually, legally Tristan.

But Anna never goes away, does she? The reminders of Anna are everywhere. I open the coat closet and there's her letter jacket from marching band with *Anna* embroidered on the front. Every time I reach into my desk drawer for a pen, I see *Anna's* first driver's permit, with long hair and thick dark eye liner, frowning for the camera. And in my briefcase is the cardboard "mousepad" that she made for me when she was about six. It's heart-shaped, white copy paper glued on cardboard, with the handwriting of six-year-old wishing me "merry X-mas Mom Love Anna" in blue ink next to a drawing of a reindeer and a Christmas tree. On the back: "Hand crafted by Anna."

And there are so many Christmas tree ornaments with her name, *Anna*.

What happens to *Anna* the name when Anna the girl becomes *Tristan* the boy? The transgender community has an answer for that. They call the birth name, the one that the parents agonized over, the *deadname*. Deadname: the very thought is one of the few things in this world that leaves me speechless.

CHAPTER 16

THE SEASON

Every new beginning comes from some other beginning's end.

~Lucius Annaeus Seneca

A few months after Tristan moved into the apartment, it was time to get ready for the second Christmas *after* (after the transgender announcement). During the previous Christmas, the first Christmas *after*, this was all very new for us. Anna was still Anna (although Lucas was the temporary name of choice). Wondering why this is relevant? Why is this even a thing? Well, it's a thing because Christmas brings with it Christmas cards, and Christmas cards are very much a *thing* in our household. To be precise, Christmas cards with a group photo of the entire family are THE thing, and that thing is non-negotiable.

Every year, sometime around Thanksgiving, we gather, the six of us (preferably in front of our newly decorated Christmas tree) for the photo of the year. Sometimes there's a boyfriend or girlfriend hanging around the house who takes the photo, or sometimes we pull in a neighbor. It's always the same scenario; at least one of the kids absolutely doesn't want to be there and is quite vocal about that, at least three kids take turns screwing up the picture, at least one parent loses their shit halfway through the photo session, and the poor boyfriend/girlfriend/neighbor who got tricked into taking the photo thinks we're all a bunch of crazies. Every year we'd mail close to two hundred of these photo cards (which seems crazy in itself since I'm pretty sure I don't even know two hundred people). This had been going on for twenty-eight years by the second Christmas after. Twenty-eight years of Mom and Dad plus one kid, then two kids, then three kids, then four. And not once in twenty-eight years had one of those kids (or Mom or Dad for that matter) had a different name than the name they had the last year.

Until the second Christmas *after*. This was the Christmas where Anna was out, and Tristan was in. Anna, in past Christmas card photos, had looked very "girly." Tristan looked very "not girly." And then there was the name thing. Sure, some people knew our situation already, but only a handful. How do you tell two hundred people (many more than that since technically most cards went to more than one person at a time; Christmas cards really are more of a household thing, aren't they?) that there is no longer an Anna in the lineup?

There was only one solution: the dreaded Christmas letter. Can you tell I'm not a fan? I do typically find Christmas letters amusing, since they're filled with all of the glorious accomplishments of the past year and none of the mess—and when you know for a fact that the accomplishments weren't nearly as glorious and that the left out messes were really messed up, that can be amusing in a twisted sort of way.

But I'm getting off track again. So, the challenge was to write a Christmas letter that didn't imply false gloriousness (is that a word?) yet neither denied nor emphasized the messiness. Oh, and don't forget the pronouns; the Christmas letter could contain NO pronouns. Because, as I said a while back, those pronouns are a bitch. And the best part of it all—the task of writing this non-glorious, limited-messiness, pronoun-less Christmas letter was all mine!

I chose a "year in review" format, with each member of the family getting a couple of lines to explain what they were doing and where they were doing it. There was not a pronoun to be found in the entire letter. Not one. Tristan's lines were exactly this:

> **Tristan:** 18, (formerly known as Anna, had a legal name
> change this year) earned state and national EMT
> certification and is now training to be a paramedic

Every single one of us, pets included, had a similar pronounless blip. Mission accomplished.

THE CHRISTMAS STOCKINGS

Our family has a weird Christmas stocking thing. It all started the first year Curt and I dated.

A little background would probably help. When I was a child my mother was at a department store just before Christmas, and there was a display model of a Christmas stocking kit that had MY name on it, spelled exactly as I spell it (which isn't how most people spell it; I'm Patti with an "i" not a "y"). Somehow my mom convinced the store clerk to sell her the ready-made sample rather than the kit. It's a beautiful felt stocking with sequins and an embroidered kitten on a felt and sequin rug next to a felt and sequin fireplace. You get the picture.

The first Christmas that Curt and I dated I had the brilliant idea to make a similar stocking for him. Off I went a few weeks before Christmas to buy the kit, and then grossly underestimated the amount of time said stocking would take to complete. But it was finished just in time for Christmas morning when he arrived at my parent's house to open gifts. (I actually never went to bed on Christmas Eve that year, but you do what you need to do to get the job done.) He picked up the stocking for what I was certain would be gushing admiration—then he turned it upside down to dump the candy bars out and see what else was inside. My eighty-seven hours of felt/sequin/embroider were second to a Snickers bar. Let's just say that he was educated in stocking etiquette that day and we all lived to tell the tale and laugh about it every year.

The felted/sequined/embroidered stockings became my thing, and I made one for each child with their name embroidered on top. Lovingly made by mom. They're stored in a special box in my closet. If the house catches fire I'm grabbing that box, 'cause there's a lot of love in there.

By the second Christmas *after*, when Tristan had moved out and was officially/legally Tristan and not Anna, it was time for a monumental stocking decision. I could not face making another one. I'm too old, and too tired (my grandchildren will definitely not be getting felted/sequined/embroidered stockings unless someone else makes them). Solution? My friend with an embroidery machine embroidered *Tristan* on a lovely gold-trimmed ribbon which I then sewed over the red embroidered *Anna* at the top of the stocking. I think it made Tristan happy; for me it was actually much harder than spending eighty-seven hours making a new one.

CHAPTER 17

THE LETTERS

I gave birth to you but you came with no instructions. All I knew was that I loved you long before I saw you. I know I made some mistakes and I am sorry. But I was doing the best I could with what I knew. Everything I did for you, I did from love. You are my child, my life, and my dreams for tomorrow. I will always love you and there is nothing that could ever destroy my love for you.

~ Amir Ahmed

The second Christmas *after* was over in a flash, and the new year brought with it a new semester of school for Tristan. She was fully involved in paramedic training but had no interest in working in that field. She continued to work at Starbucks instead. At this point we're about eighteen months after her transgender announcement. I'd like to say that we were all adjusting nicely to our new normal, but that would be a total lie.

Tristan was looking more male than ever, and I was struggling with it. The hormones were definitely doing their job. But the hormones weren't enough for Tristan anymore. Once again, it was time to up the game. Tristan had very little interaction with me or Curt, but when she did it was usually about only one thing—top surgery. She had met with a plastic surgeon who had agreed to perform the surgery. Top surgery is exactly what it sounds like: breast removal. I should have seen this coming, realized that this was inevitable, but it still blindsided me. I had friends who had lost their breasts to cancer, and now my eighteen-year-old daughter (yes, in my mind she's still my daughter) wants to cut off her two healthy breasts. And, she has found a plastic surgeon who will perform a mastectomy without hesitation. Who was this quack, I wanted to know? Tristan refused to tell me his/her name. She'd even paid for the initial visit in cash rather than run it through insurance to be certain that I wouldn't be able to find out who the doctor was. She really does think of everything. I'm not sure what she thought I'd do if I found out the name, but I'm sure she wasn't taking any chances after the episode with the endocrinologist a few months back.

By now Tristan was avoiding me like the plague, except when there was something she wanted/needed (those two are easily confused, aren't they?). Right now, she wanted three things:

1. For me (and Curt) to support her decision to have her breasts removed—at age eighteen.

2. For me to nurse her through her recovery period (which she estimated to be two weeks, which I thought was ridiculously underestimated).

3. For us to allow her to have our insurance company pay for the surgery.

Remember when we were pre-testosterone and Tristan was constantly pounding us because all she wanted was to start the testosterone trial? Every conversation, every moment we were together revolved around her wanting to begin a testosterone trial. She was relentless. Well, her new passion was top surgery. At age eighteen. Once again, she was a dog with a bone, and she wasn't letting go.

Any other communication between me and Tristan for the next few months consisted of things like this:

• She wanted a new phone, didn't like the way hers was acting. I suggested a trip to the phone store to see if they could fix it under our warranty. She'd say that it couldn't be fixed and that I was treating her like a complete idiot. *And, by the way, she really needed me to support her top surgery.*

• She broke her retainer. Used broken phone to tell me that she didn't have time to make an orthodontic appointment, took time to go over her entire week's schedule with me so that I could make the appointment. *Top surgery somehow worked into the conversation.*

• She still wanted a new phone. Used supposedly broken phone to tell me that if I don't get her a new phone then she will get her own phone plan. I still eagerly await that day.

• I'd send her photos of Caly doing something particularly adorable. She'd respond appropriately and then ask if we wanted to take her out to dinner.

• She broke her retainer, again. Same resolution as above, *top surgery made the conversation.*

• She'd send me photos of Freyja (her cat) doing something particularly adorable. I'd respond appropriately and then ask if she'd like to come to the house for dinner.

• I'd send photos of new health insurance card (to broken phone which still seemed to not be broken). Card had the name "Anna Marie." Tristan complained that name was incorrect, yet I had no paperwork showing corrected legal name. Tristan sends scan of legal name change document and new driver's license using broken phone (which is still not broken). *Reminds me not to try and dissuade her from top surgery.*

• She wanted to go shopping for clothes. Texted me using broken phone.

• I texted broken phone to see if she'd ever filed legal name-change paperwork with insurance company. She answered no.

• I let her know that, after a nine month wait, Paula (the dream therapist, my number one pick) had openings and was awaiting her call. She could keep James and add Paula. The answer was a big fat "NO." *And, by the way, James supports the top surgery.*

• She needs a dermatologist, and I don't find the name of mine quickly enough. She uses the still-broken phone to tell me that she " . . . literally might have cancer so I hope you tried to find the dermatologist's stupid name. Because if it is cancer, and it very well might be, you're gonna feel like shit if it's worse than it could've been because you wouldn't get me her name." Gave her the name, and never heard another word about it so I'm assuming it wasn't terminal.

• She wants more money, and if I won't give it to her she'll ask her grandparents. I suggest she work more hours since she is an adult and that's what adults do when they want more money. She suggests that she'll get a credit card and go into deep debt instead. *She needs all of the money she can get in case she has to pay for her top surgery out of pocket.*

That was our life, until the two-year anniversary of the transgender announcement. By now she had learned that Starbucks would pay for her bachelor's degree, and she knew that there was no way she could continue the paramedic training, work, and pursue a B.S., so she made a very grown-up decision to put the paramedic training on hold in order to pursue the B.S. But there was some lag time between the time when the paramedic training stopped and the bachelor's coursework began. Tristan had a lot more time on her hands since there was no schoolwork for a few months, which gave her plenty of time to focus on top surgery.

While the testosterone trial was certainly hard for me to go along with (perhaps that's an understatement), this top surgery was unbearable. I still wasn't convinced (not even close) that Tristan was truly transgender. I didn't believe that the inordinate amount of therapy had even scratched the surface of whatever the real issue was. And there was no way on God's green earth that I was going to stand by and watch quietly as she allowed some quack plastic surgeon to cut off her breasts. I told her in no uncertain terms that I considered it mutilation of her body, and I would not support it. I did offer a compromise; I told her that if she waited until age twenty-five and still wanted to have the top surgery then she could do so with my full support—and my insurance. Once again, there was not enough "hell no" in HELL NO to convey her rejection of that idea. At that point I let her know that if she did try to have the top surgery then she would do so without using my health insurance coverage. That obviously went over like a lead balloon.

She came to us (me and Curt) just before her nineteenth birthday with new ammunition, the target being those three things she wanted from us so desperately: our emotional support, physical care, and insurance money for her top surgery. Her ammo of choice as she went in for the kill? Two letters, one from the Shrink (Dr. Davidson, the psychiatrist who had given Tristan seventeen minutes of psychotherapy and a whole lot of prescriptions over the last twelve months) and one from Tristan herself. She dropped these letters off for us at our house one afternoon while we weren't home. Both were addressed to me and Curt, both were written to make a plea for Tristan's top surgery, and one was written quite well.

Tristan's letter was informative and polite. She let us know that she was planning for the top surgery and was hoping for our support—emotional and financial. She wanted to know how we planned to handle the insurance coverage, and if she should make arrangements to get her own health insurance (this will take a turn shortly). Dr. Davidson's letter implored us to reconsider our stance on the health insurance matter, and assured us that she could recommend a top-notch plastic surgeon to perform the mastectomy (wonderful, another plastic surgeon who is eager to remove the breasts of a teenager). She let us know that she was confident that Tristan would greatly benefit from the surgery, and that HE (Dr. Davidson was/is a whiz at the pronouns) was unwilling to go through with the surgery unless HE knew that we would not drop HIM from our health insurance.

I was a little confused by this, as Tristan's letter had said that she was planning to go through with the surgery no matter what, while Dr. Davidson said that Tristan was unwilling to go through with it unless she could use our insurance. However, that was the least of my worries with Dr. Davidson's letter. What bothered me most about Dr. Davidson's letter was the quality, not the content. Her letter, all half-page of it, contained one completely wrong word, one misspelling, four run-on sentences, a missed hyphen, and one unnecessary comma. Me being petty? *Probably.* Somebody thinks she's the grammar police? *Maybe.* Mama concerned that this medical doctor (who had written to inform me that she'd observed my child and could assure me that this surgery was the right course of action in this case) had paid so little attention to detail that she missed eight errors in one short letter? *Absolutely!*

Did I think that Tristan would actually go through with top surgery? Not really, at least not anytime soon. Her letter was written in August, and in it she said that she was planning for the surgery in December. I just didn't see that as a viable time frame. As much as I wanted to destroy those letters and pretend like I never saw them, I knew that I needed to put on my big-girl pants and deal with it. It was time for a plan. Curt and I discussed our options (which were clearly limited: support top surgery or don't) and decided that we needed to know more. And we needed Tristan to know more. I had a feeling that Tristan looked at top surgery as a solution to all her problems and wasn't seeing it for what it really was—a cosmetic change.

THE SOCIAL MEDIA

I admire people with perfect children, honestly, I do. They're out there, and I know this because I see them on social media every time I log in. We all see them, don't we? Perfect families with perfect parents and perfect children. Social media would never lie, right? And, in my mind, their perfection magnifies my imperfection. I wasn't a perfect child, nor was I a perfect teenager, and I'll never be a perfect parent. But I try. And I fail. I say the wrong things, I do the wrong things, and then I start all over again the next day convinced that I will do better. I try. And I fail. I fail because I, like those objects of my social media envy, will never be perfect—no matter how much I try.

About two years *after,* after Anna left and Tristan came, I joined a social media group that was formed to support parents of transgender children. This was a closed group; to be accepted you needed to ask permission and tell the administrator why you wanted/needed to be in this group. It was designed to be a "no judgement zone," which was awesome because judgement was the last thing I needed.

Once I was accepted into the group, I eased myself in. I basically stalked other people's posts, making the occasional comment ("I feel you; we're in the same boat" or something similar) or just hitting the "like" button. I'm not sure what I expected from this group, but I was shocked at what I read. There were certainly some parents like me, parents who were shocked when their child announced out of the blue that they were transgender, but we were definitely in the minority. And there were the others, the majority, the ones who sounded like having their child announce they were transgender was the equivalent of telling them they were going to 7-11 to get a Slurpee.

"Thanks so much for adding me to this group! My son told us yesterday that he's transgender! Isn't that wonderful! We're so thrilled! Yesterday we had a beautiful daughter named Tiffany and today we have a handsome son named Bruce! We can't wait to go to the barber shop today to get Bruce a proper haircut then off to the courthouse to get that name-change ball rolling. He's told us that he still LOVES to wear makeup, and he may still wear dresses from time to time, but he's totally male otherwise. I must say we were totally surprised, but YEAH! I can't wait to tell the grand-parents!"

And there were the posts that shocked me most, the ones by parents of young children, toddlers even, who jumped on the trans-gender bandwagon with reckless abandon before their child was even potty trained.

"I'm so glad I found this group; I'm not sure how I'd go on without it. I have three daughters in elementary school and a twenty-two-month-old son. Four months ago, when he was eighteen months old, little Johnny was playing with his sister when he looked at me with his sweet little smile and said, 'Me a girl, too.' I'd never heard him say that before! If it weren't for this group, I'm not sure I would have known what to do! Luckily, I was prepared to meet this head on. I

immediately stopped using ANY male pronouns with
Johnny, and I made sure he knew that it was ok if he wanted
to wear girl clothes and have us call him a girl name. Thank
you, thank you to all of you for your support. Now little
Johnny can grow up to be the girl he should have been all
along."

I've exaggerated the tone a little in those two posts, but only the
tone and not the message. The message in each one is exactly as
the "poster" relayed it; only the names have been changed. They
both concern me deeply, for different reasons. The first mom's post
gave me emotional whiplash. I just cannot imagine that in just
twenty-four hours she's said goodbye to Tiffany, hello to Bruce, and
is basically dancing a jig. How can anyone adjust to something so
life altering so quickly?

The second one is just so disturbing. I've raised four children,
and there are countless other young people in my life that I've
known since their birth. And I can say with complete confidence
that every toddler I've ever know has, at some point, been confused
about Gender 101. Johnny has three sisters. Johnny learns from
mom and dad that Jenny is a girl, Julie is a girl, and mommy is a
girl. Johnny is a boy, and daddy is a boy. Johnny is a boy like daddy.
I wonder, just for kicks and giggles, what would have happened to
little Johnny if mom had said, "No, Johnny is a boy like daddy.
Jenny, Julie and Janie are girls like mommy." Maybe Johnny would
have still grown up to be a transgender MTF (male to female), who
knows. But I'm convinced that giving up male pronouns and
offering your male toddler his choice of girl clothes and a girl name
because he utters "me a girl" one time may just be one of the best
examples of insanity I've ever heard.

I realize that there's no room for judgement, and I'm really
trying not to judge. I'm just confused. And concerned. And I feel
pain for these people. They're really my people, aren't they? We're
all trying to figure it out, and criticism isn't what any of us need. A
friend told me not long ago that she was asked by another friend

how she'd feel if her child came to her and said they were gay? Her answer: *I'm not sure I'd feel anything, if he's gay he's gay. No big deal.* Then he asked her how she'd feel if her child came to her and said they were transgender. Her answer: *That's different. I don't know how I'd feel. That's so new, it's so confusing. I just don't think I'd understand.* Her answer nails it.

This whole transgender world is new, it's confusing, and it's hard to understand. How do you know your five-year-old boy isn't simply feminine or perhaps gay rather than give him a label of transgender? There are plenty of cisgender (someone whose gender identity is that of their birth gender—born a female and identifies as a female, or born a male and identifies as a male) men/women who have feminine/masculine characteristics as well without being gay or transgender. I just wonder if sometimes we're too quick to label.

CHAPTER 18

THE IMPASSE

Grief, I've learned, is really just love. It's all the love you want to give but cannot. All of that unspent love gathers in the corners of your eyes, the lump in your throat, and in the hollow part of your chest. Grief is just love with no place to go.

~ Jamie Anderson

Tristan's a September baby, so August is usually filled with birthday plans for the big event. In 2019, it was quite different. Instead of planning her nineteenth birthday celebration, Curt and I were planning how to deal with the letters—one from Tristan, and one from Dr. Flash.

Here's what I knew I had to work with:

- Trying to ignore the topic of top surgery or delaying the

conversation was nonsensical, so I needed to meet it head-on ASAP.

- Any conversation with Tristan about this was going to get really ugly really quickly unless I was in complete agreement with whatever she wanted.

I knew with complete certainty how this scenario would play out: we'd sit down together, agree to discuss this whole top surgery thing like rational people, then we'd all lose it and end up back to square one. Solution? Meet in a neutral place. No raised voices, no slammed doors, just conversation—questions and answers. Tristan wasn't a fan of the neutral-place idea, but she agreed. We (me, Curt, Tristan) met at a local coffee shop (not Starbucks), and I came prepared with my list of questions and thoughts. After we exchanged pleasantries and all agreed that this was simply a discussion, and that we would all play nice, it went something like this:

- Question: What's the recovery time look like for this type of surgery, and who will help you with your recovery?
- *Answer: Two weeks maybe, I'm not sure. I don't know who'll help.*
- Question: Your letter mentioned that you've made arrangements to cover your income while you're out of work for the recovery period. What arrangements are those?
- *Answer: I'm going to get the money from Andrew* (brother number two, who at this point in time had graduated from college and was not yet earning an income).
- Question: What's the total cost of the surgery?
- *Answer: I don't know.*
- Question: You've asked us to allow you to use our health insurance plan to pay for it. We have several thousand dollars left to meet our deductible, then there's a twenty

percent co-pay. If we allow you to use our health
insurance plan to pay for the surgery, how will you pay
for the deductible and co-pay?
- *Answer: I don't know.*
- Question: You've said that Starbucks has great health
insurance, and that you'll eventually get health
insurance through them. What does that look like?
- *Answer: Right now, I have a seven-hundred-dollar deductible*
and a thirty percent co-pay. I pay a hundred and seventy-five
dollars every month for it.

(Side note: in an interesting turn of events, suddenly Tristan has
her own health insurance. I was unaware. Dr. Davidson was clearly
unaware as well, since her letter indicated that lack of insurance
coverage was the only thing standing in the way of Tristan going
forward with the surgery.)

- Question: You just said that you pay a hundred and
seventy-five dollars a month for health insurance. When
did this happen?
- *Answer: Months ago, I told you.*
- C: (C is for comment, since the list of questions went out
the window at that point.) No, you didn't tell me. Now I
understand why our insurance company keeps sending
me letters demanding to know who our second health
insurance carrier is. I keep filling out the forms and
sending them back telling them to quit harassing me
because none of us have additional health insurance.
Oh My God, have I committed insurance fraud?
- *Answer: Oh My God, Mom, that's not insurance fraud.*

The conversation pretty much went downhill from there. It was
clear that in her letter Dr. Davidson had been quick to try and
school me on the absolute necessity (in her opinion) for the top
surgery, but no one had taken the time to school Tristan about the

nuts and bolts (or the dollars and cents) of the whole thing. Top surgery is major surgery, and carries all of the risks you would expect: reactions to anesthesia, blood clots, infection.

Tristan had no clue that top surgery would cost about $10,000 for the surgeon's fee (according to the Healthline.com), then there are facility fees, anesthesiologist fees, $20-per-pill Tylenol fees, and the list goes on. Fun fact: a 2019 businessinsider.com report estimated that there are 1.4 million transgender individuals living in the U.S., and that some spend as much as $100,000 on surgeries to align their bodies with their gender identities. There's top surgery, bottom surgery, facial and body hair removal surgery, and the list goes on.

I was annoyed about the insurance; Tristan was annoyed because we didn't surprise her with unconditional emotional and financial support for the upcoming top surgery. The meeting ended much like it started, with everyone tense and upset. We walked Tristan to her car, and the rage set in. In classic Tristan fashion, she threw a fit in the parking lot. She hadn't gotten what she wanted, and she was plenty pissed off about it.

And then it hit me. This was less about insurance and more about control. She had insurance, good insurance, but she didn't want to use her insurance. She wanted to use ours. And frankly, I didn't think she even wanted to go through with the surgery. Tristan is a planner and a researcher. Her attention to detail is beyond impressive. There's no way that she would make a plan for top surgery until she knew exactly what it involved and what it costs. She just wanted to see how far she could push. She'd gone so far down the road that she couldn't turn back, so she just kept going. Top surgery was the next logical step.

The next few days were a blur of tears and guilt. How do you support your child without compromising your beliefs? I don't mean just religious beliefs, although they certainly play a part. (I believe that God loves Tristan as much as He loved Anna, and that He put her on this earth to do amazing things with her life, whether she's transgender, cisgender, or whatever else she may be.)

It's when you believe with all of your heart that your child has made the wrong choices for the wrong reasons. It's when you see it, you get it, but they don't, and there's not a thing you can do to help. You see that there's a piece missing to this whole puzzle, but you can't find it no matter how hard you try. And the people who are supposed to help you look (the Debras, and the Jameses, and Dr. Davidsons) just flat out aren't looking; they don't want to solve the puzzle because for them it's not about the solution. It's just too hard when you love them, but you don't agree with their choices and decisions, and yet they equate agreeing with acceptance and love. "If you don't agree with me, then you don't accept me, and you certainly don't love me."

Tristan had her own agenda over the next few days. She sent us more emails than I could keep up with. She sent information about her Starbucks health insurance plan, and she sent LOTS of links to websites that were intended to educate me (and Curt) on all things transgender related. In fact, she sent sixty-three links in less than twenty-four hours. SIXTY-THREE. There were twelve links for articles on the *similarity of the neuroanatomy of transgender and cisgender individuals* (causing major confusion on my part since I'm quite sure I have no idea what that means) to explain why being transgender is a *natural phenomenon* (her words). There were thirty-seven links to articles on studies about gender dysphoria and the brain. Six of the links were to articles dealing with post-transition (after a person has transitioned to a different gender). Eight of the links were to general transgender articles. Once again, I was exhausted and overwhelmed by the whole thing.

WE ARE ELEVEN

Curt and I have been married for a really long time, almost thirty-three years at this point. We had a big celebration for our thirtieth wedding anniversary a few years ago; we renewed our vows and then had a big dinner party at a nice restaurant. We thought that it would be appropriate for us to say a few words to thank the thirty-five or so friends and family who had joined us, and I nominated Curt for the task. I had no idea what he was planning to say; when I asked, he just told me that he had it under control. How do you drive a control freak crazy? Tell her that you have it all under control and refuse to elaborate. So, the time came for a toast; we stood up together for Curt to thank the crowd. He thanked them, and then he told a story. Actually, he told a private story, a story that was our little secret. (Nothing scandalous; it was only a secret because, up to that point, there had been no reason to share it.) But, since he shared it with all of our friends, I'll share it here. Our secret is this: we call ourselves, the two of us, *Team Eleven*. What in the hell does that mean, you may ask? Let me explain.

One Sunday at church years ago the minister preached about relationships, and specifically how you prioritize the relationships you have with the people in your life. The more important they are to you, the higher the priority, so the lower the number. (Example: the mailman might not be as important to you, so maybe he's number seven hundred and fourteen in your life while the Amazon delivery guy [soooo important, at least to me] might be number twelve; your kids, however, likely have single digits on your priority list.) The minister's point was to have each of us think about the people in our own lives and figure out where they all fit. Who are our priorities?

It seems pretty simple on the surface, but I think that a lot of people lose sight of who's really most important to them. If you really think about it, it's a question that we should each ask ourselves. After church Curt and I discussed it quite a bit, and the result of our analysis was this; we truly live our lives as each other's number one. To us that simply means that we each put the other first, although it may mean something else to you. Since he's my number one, and I'm his number one, we came up with Team Eleven. I've oversimplified a bit, but the reality is that not all married couples are truly each other's number one. Marriage is hard, parenting is hard; both bring stress and conflict no matter what you do to avoid it. Stress can certainly damage any relationship; marriage is no exception. Tristan's "coming out" as transgender has certainly been stressful on both of us. I'd be lying if I said otherwise. But Team Eleven handles the stress so that Patti and Curt don't need to handle it alone. While we haven't always agreed on everything one hundred percent, we've handled everything one hundred percent together. That's Team Eleven.

CHAPTER 19

THE REALITY

We must accept finite disappointment but never lose infinite hope.

~ Martin Luther King, Jr.

———————

To say that my relationship with Tristan went from bad to worse is an understatement. It had actually gone from bad to intolerable. Tristan wasn't living at home, was barely speaking to me, and yet she consumed my life. (Personal opinion here: unless your child suffers from a terminal illness, you are NOT in a healthy situation if your child consumes your every thought.)

Every waking moment was spent thinking about her, worrying about her, wanting to reach out to her and help her, to sit on the couch and hold her and hug her and keep hugging her until she said *Mom, let go of me*. But I wanted to hug Anna, and Anna was gone. I was distracted at home; I was distracted at work. I wasn't doing anything well, and I felt lost.

I really have no idea why Tristan thought that dropping off a couple of letters at the house and meeting in a coffee shop to chat would suddenly make us think *Oh, silly us, we should definitely do a complete about-face and jump on board for her top surgery. Why didn't we see the logic in this before now? After all, she is almost nineteen, nineteen-year-olds never change their minds about anything, and are fully emotionally equipped to make irreparable life-altering decisions.*

But apparently, she did think just that because after our little chat (and the ensuing onslaught of sixty-three emails with their never-ending links to all things transgender) it was game-on for Tristan. She would not stop until she won. Our battle had turned into a war, and she was armed with new ammunition which she fired through another round of endless emails. The day we met at the coffee shop to discuss the top surgery (after the letters) she had misinterpreted our asking questions as being an offer of support. When our Q&A session ended without that support it blew her mind. And so began an all-new email campaign. Curt was the target of most of her emails, likely because she enjoys engaging people (she's really quite good at debate) and Curt is always happy to engage when presented with the opportunity. The two of them are very much alike in that, although Curt (as he gets older) enjoys a healthy exchange of ideas while Tristan enjoys the opportunity to bring out her verbal hammer and pound away. I'd like to think that age has something to do with the way those two handle their differences, similar as they are; she brings the passion of youth to every disagreement while he balances that passion with a more mellow stance that comes with age—and exhaustion.

Since none of the medical doctors who were pushing her to have top surgery had actually taken time to discuss the practical and financial issues that are part of this, Curt and I had tried to help Tristan understand that adult decisions require adult information, and she needed all of the information in order to make an informed and intelligent decision. Tristan sent an email detailing her health insurance plan—co-pays, deductibles, in network vs. out of network, adult stuff. Curt responded with a breakdown of the numbers in hopes of enlightening her as to the financial ramifications of what would be a very costly procedure. Tristan would have none of it. She didn't care about the finances. As far as she was concerned that was something to think about another day, like after the surgery was done. He was completely honest with her that neither he nor I could support her decision to have top surgery at such a young age. He and I both saw a beautiful, brilliant young lady who, for reasons that completely alluded us, seemed to despise herself. She didn't like who she was, and she simply wanted to be someone else. She had never, until the day in the car on the winding road, given any indication that she was a male trapped in a female body. Never. Nothing. It was like someone flipped a switch; one day I was telling her to lighten up on the eye shadow and put on a tank top because her V-neck t-shirt was showing too much cleavage, and the next day she's telling us that she's ALWAYS felt like a male. Curt and I were "willfully ignorant" and making up "bullshit excuses" to avoid accepting (her) reality. She was quite clear that we did not love her. She claimed that her mental health was much improved as long as she wasn't around us, and that being away from us allowed her to, in fact, finally love herself. We (Curt and I) were the issue, the only issue. Oh, and we were dimwits (that's a quote). Next came the infamous emails with their sixty-three links to articles that were certain to convince us that you can, indeed, flip a switch and go from female to male in no time flat.

I've never in my life met a person who responds positively to being constantly cursed and berated. However, I live in reality so I know that everyone loses their temper sometimes, and that everyone deserves a pass from time to time when they lose their cool and have a meltdown. I firmly believe that you will never convince someone to change their mind/opinion/stance by screaming at them and insulting them. I'm no psychologist, but I know that it just doesn't work that way. But by now the Tristan meltdowns were out of control. To the best of my knowledge, Curt and I were the only target. For months we had had minimal interaction with her, but what interaction we did have with her was unbearable. We could do nothing right, and she was more than happy to point that out at every opportunity. Finally, we realized that Tristan was absolutely right. Tristan was right, we were dimwits. We were dimwits for allowing her to treat us the way she did. She cursed us, she berated us, she insulted us, and we allowed it. The question was why? Why in the world would two seemingly intelligent people (believe it or not, we really aren't dimwits) tolerate this crap? And then it dawned on us—we didn't have to tolerate it at all. We would never have allowed anyone else to treat us that way, so why was Tristan allowed to? She was legally an adult, living on her own (with our financial support, of course), and she was choosing to treat us like absolute dirt. And we had chosen to accept it. That was a harsh reality, but we had to face or it we'd never be able to fix it. So, now what? That was the hardest part. I remember years ago when "tough love" was the big parent-speak. Over-tolerant parents were boldly requiring their (usually adult) children to accept personal responsibility. No more mommy and daddy coming to the rescue and bailing them out of their messes. Curt and I decided it was time for our own version of tough love. Maybe in our case it was more "firm love" than tough love. All we knew was that we couldn't go on anymore with things the way they were, and it was up to us to redefine our relationship with Tristan. The tail would no longer wag the dog.

There's one key piece of this whole messy puzzle that needs to be singled out. Believe it or not, by now the issues we were having had little to do with Tristan's chosen transgender lifestyle. As Curt very simply pointed out in one of their many email exchanges, this was not at all a transgender thing, this was a nice person thing. And Tristan, at least when she was with us, was behaving like anything but a nice person.

Parent/child relationships should not need recreating or redefining, but sometimes they do, and it's not easy. It's heart wrenching, it's tearful, it stinks, but sometimes it's the only choice you have. When Tristan was Anna and was studying martial arts, she did some sparring competitions. Sometimes an opponent would "tap out." In case you don't know martial arts slang, tapping out means to "tap" on the floor to indicate that you've had enough, that you're done with the round and can't go on. Curt and I decided it was time to tap out.

CHILDREN ARE CHALLENGES

I remember years ago having a conversation with our pediatrician. We were talking about how differently some kids behave when they're at school versus when they're at home. Some kids behave better at home than at school, and some are the opposite. At the time I was discussing one of my older children, and I was telling him how hard it was for me to believe that this child's teachers had zero behavioral issues, no complaints at all. Home, however, was a different story. This particular child of mine was a challenge (or so I thought that said child was a challenge; that was before Anna became Tristan and I learned what a real challenge was).

This was a good kid with a heart of gold and a mission in life to find out exactly what it would take to send me over the edge. This one put the "A" in attitude. I didn't get it: great at school, mini wrecking ball at home. The pediatrician wasn't surprised at all. His explanation for why some kids behave so well at school and so crummy at home? Because home is safe, it's the place where they can let it out, no matter what "it" is, and they know that their parents will love them no matter what. No matter how crazy they make you, no matter what they do, they're still your kid and you'll still love them. And the pediatrician was right; I loved that mini wrecking ball all of those years ago despite the fact that I was constantly teetering on the edge of sanity. But I only teetered; I never went over the edge.

And I won't go over the edge with Tristan, either, although I often feel like the slightest tap could send me right over. I hope that one day Tristan sees me as two things: 1) a mama who was strong enough to never go over the edge, no matter how close she got, and 2) a mama who loved her no matter what.

CHAPTER 20

THE ESTRANGEMENT

I've got some issues that nobody can see
And all of these emotions are pouring out of me
I bring them to the light for you
It's only right
This is the soundtrack to my life

~ Kid Cudi in *Soundtrack to My Life*

It was almost two years to the day since the car ride down the winding road that I hate so much now. The name change I could handle, and the gender transition I would be able to adjust to in time. Hell, I might even be able to handle the pronouns one day. But the vile attitude and complete disrespect were more than I could deal with. Firm love was the only choice. Have I made it sound easy? Well, it wasn't.

Two years ago, I woke up one morning with a daughter named Anna, a daughter that I'd loved for seventeen years. When I went to bed that night, Anna was gone. But she wasn't really gone, she just wasn't there—if that makes sense. This person was there in her place, this person that looked like Anna, sounded like Anna, but insisted that she wasn't Anna anymore. I'd spent the last two years searching for Anna, hoping she'd come back. But this new person was my roadblock; she wasn't letting Anna through. And I couldn't mourn Anna, because how do you mourn someone who's not there anymore, yet she's not gone either?

There's a saying that when God closes a door, He opens a window. For me the door was nailed shut and the window was stuck. This was parental hell of a type that I never knew existed. What's the emotion that lies in the middle of joy and mourning? Is it existing? If it's existing then that's what I was doing, and I was barely doing it. I kept telling myself, "At least she's here. It could be so much worse." And yes, it could have been so much worse. I have friends, too many friends, who have suffered the unbearable loss of a child. My loss was minuscule in comparison. My child was alive on this earth and for that I was, and still am, grateful beyond words. But the truth here is that, as a mother, I needed to mourn. My family had changed, and it would never be the same. Someone I loved was gone. I couldn't mourn the child, the child who wasn't there yet wasn't gone. I needed to mourn the family that I used to have, the one that would never be the same again. Yet I couldn't. I couldn't mourn because it wasn't right. How dare I mourn when others had it so much worse. Mourning wasn't an option. But continuing on as we had been for so many months wasn't an option either.

Since our communication with Tristan was now relegated to email, Curt sent her an email to let her know that we'd had enough. One of us had to send it, and he volunteered to send the email since he knew that I likely couldn't handle it. Here's what it said, in a nutshell:

- Curt and I had discussed this situation and were in complete agreement as to how to go forward.

- Tristan's transgender lifestyle wasn't the issue. Transgender people have the same capacity to be nice that cisgender people have; her unkind behavior toward us was a decision far removed from her transgender lifestyle.
- We had no intention of seeing her spiral into poverty. There was no way that she could support herself with only her part-time Starbucks job. Since we were currently providing Tristan with a fairly substantial monthly allowance since she was still in school at this point, we agreed to increase the monthly amount and continue it for eighteen months. This would allow her to finish the paramedic program and get established in a full-time job.
- Tristan would now need to become financially responsible (with the help of the monthly allowance from us) for everything: tuition, books, car insurance, rent, you name it. We had worked out a budget that would cover everything and even allow her to start a rainy-day fund to give her a little cushion. She'd need to spend wisely and save wisely.
- The car she drove would be put in her name and would become her responsibility.
- She had her own health insurance, so she'd come off of ours the following month.
- She could stay on our cell phone service plan. I have no idea why we decided this, but it seemed logical at the time. I think the cheapskate in me couldn't bear to see her pay the cell phone company for an individual plan.

In essence, we were firm-loving her into adulthood with all of its glory and accompanying responsibilities (minus the cell phone thing). But we knew Tristan. And we knew that we'd be back to the same old same old as soon as you could say *I need fifty-dollars because there was this commercial on TV with a really sad-looking cat and I sent them money and now I can't pay my rent.* So, we needed to set boundaries; after all what's firm love without boundaries? The boundaries were pretty tight:

- Don't contact us.
- Don't come to the house.
- This may last weeks, months, or years, but it will last as long as it needs to.

Let's step back a little. The day that Tristan told me she was transgender she immediately followed by telling me that she was expecting to be kicked out of the house. She'd actually made plans to move in with her friend Krystal's family since she was certain that I'd tell her to pack up her bags and hit the road. I was actually a little taken back by her sense of disappointment when that didn't happen. She'd obviously created a scenario in her head about the poor, downtrodden, transgender assigned female at birth (AFAB) who'd been abandoned by her family and forced to live off of the kindness of semi-strangers as she made her way through the cold, cruel, intolerant world. The plot was written; the characters were cast. It was a blockbuster hit in the making. It seemed to blow her mind when that didn't happen; in fact, she told me several times in the first few weeks *after* that she was really shocked that I didn't respond by blowing a gasket. (My wording, not hers. Odd term, isn't it? I know that blowing a gasket means to get really angry, but WTH does it really have to do with anything?)

Now here we were, acting out our own (modified) version of Tristan's life story, kicking Tristan to the curb. She'd already moved out and was living in her own apartment, so we obviously weren't kicking her out of the house. But we were effectively kicking her out of our lives. That's pretty painful to write; to see it in black and white feels ugly. I was beginning to wonder if this situation we found ourselves in was really her self-fulfilling prophecy. She had focused on being estranged from her family for so long that it was bound to happen. She made certain of it.

If you listen to enough self-help jargon, you'll eventually hear a phrase like this: What you focus on expands. Pretty self-explanatory, right? If you focus on the negative you'll end up with negative things; if you focus on the positive . . . Had Tristan spent so much time focusing on estrangement that she basically willed it to happen?

THE WRONG DMV

Life is funny sometimes, isn't it? You're going about the everyday business of life, like going to the DMV or something equally torturous, and out of nowhere—BAM—you're in the middle of a situation that you never expected in a million years. Such was the situation I found myself in just a week or so after the invocation of *"firm love."* Remember the part about putting the car in Tristan's name? Well, that little act required a trip to a local DMV branch. You see, the car was in both of our names, mine and Tristan's, and the objective was to change the title to her name only. Off to the DMV I went, but not to the DMV branch that I normally go to.

For some reason I was compelled beyond understanding (this sounds silly and weird, but I'm totally serious) to go to the DMV branch that I hate the most. Hate is a strong word, and I don't hate many things, but I HATE that particular branch of the DMV. It was like my car was on autopilot that day, and off it went to the most unmagical place on earth. You probably know the DMV drill; take a number, wait. Wait. Wait. There are twenty-seven customer service windows, nineteen people working at those windows, and two hundred and forty-nine customers waiting in hard molded plastic chairs.

So, there I sat, paperwork in hand, wondering exactly how it was that two hundred and forty-eight of the two hundred and forty-nine people waiting with me seemed to be coughing up a lung. My hand sanitizer and I continued to wait until they called E321, my magic number. The lady at the customer service window, Chelle, was thrilled to see me. She only had to see approximately nine hundred people over the course of the next five hours, and then she could go home. But that's not the point. The point is what Chelle said to me as she processed my paperwork.

She pulled up the information for the car on her computer, then she pulled up the information on the two owners (me and Tristan at the time). Then she looked at the title. Then she looked confused. Then she said the oddest thing to me, "I have a transgender child, too." WTF said my brain, while my mouth said something clever like, "Huh?" Now I was the one who looked confused. And she explained. She saw on the computer screen that the owners were me and someone named Tristan, but the title said me and Anna. She quickly put two and two together. We spent the next seventy-five minutes bonding at the customer service window (your tax dollars at work).

Chelle was the first person I'd met who'd gone through what I was going through and had lived to tell the tale. She'd been in the transgender trenches for about six years, and she was a wealth of insight. I had so much to ask, and she had so much to say. After about forty-five minutes when I asked if she might be questioned by her supervisor (who was by now staring a hole in her back) about the amount of time we'd spent together she told me not to worry, that if necessary she'd just explain what a pain in the ass customer I'd been and that she had done her best to send me on my way. Perfect solution, and it bought us another thirty minutes. By this point I was convinced that God had put us together (why else would I have gone to the most hated DMV I've ever known), and He clearly would want us to take our time as we bonded over tales of motherhood confusion.

When I finally left Chelle's window, we had traded email

addresses and promised to get together for a drink to support one another through the trials and tribulations of mothering a transgender child. A few days later I sent her an email. Crickets. My new BFF was gone from my life as quickly as she came into it. I wonder if she checked her spam folder. It must be in her spam folder, otherwise I'm certain that I would have heard from her. She has my phone number, too; why hasn't she called? Ever the optimist, I'm still waiting for her to return my email, or better yet, ring my phone. Chelle, you broke my heart, but it serves me right for going to the wrong DMV.

CHAPTER 21

THE CONTACT

Grief changes shape, but it never ends.

~ Keanu Reeves

The *Firm Love No Contact* thing seemed easy on the surface but was not so easy from a practical standpoint. You can't just say, "See ya," and be done with it. There are details to work out; I imagine it's a bit like separating from a spouse (pretty crappy comparison, right?). Tristan needed to figure out how to take over adult things like car insurance and personal property taxes (she'd already mastered health insurance, so we were good there). As she took over those little details, we let them go, which meant coordination. Basically, no contact wasn't really no contact. It was extremely limited contact, which was okay with me. A mama is always a mama, and mamas need contact with their babies. And Tristan will always be my baby. So, we'd work out the details via text (it was a miracle— the broken phone still managed to work), then no contact until the next detail popped up.

A few weeks after our FLNC (firm love no contact; I love acronyms) I was faced with a dilemma; it was Tristan's birthday. Before FLNC this would have meant a family meal with her favorite dish (spaghetti carbonara in case you're wondering; I make the BEST spaghetti carbonara ever), cake and ice cream, and gifts. The siblings and the grandparents show up, and the birthday kid has the option to invite friends. But this year, the first year of FLNC, there would be no massive amount of bacon for the spaghetti carbonara, no cake, nothing. I was cool as a cucumber on the outside; inside I was a mess. The morning of her birthday I sent her a text message (someone please tell me what we did before this amazing technology; did we, perhaps, talk to other people using our voices?) letting her know that I/we had paid her personal property taxes on her car (so much for adulting), had transferred some money into her bank account (FLNC obviously still allowed us to be connected via online banking) that I hoped would be used to buy something she WANTED rather than NEEDED, and that I/we hoped she had a nice day. I knew that she had spent her birthday eve with her grandparents (spaghetti carbonara and coconut cake since I was the birthday consultant rather than participant that year) and was working at Starbucks on her actual birthday. So how did I spend her birthday, her first birthday without mama? I stayed home and drank wine. Okay, don't judge me. I know that drinking wine to escape sadness is sad in itself. (Truth be told, we're not even big drinkers. We're occasional weekend social drinkers at best. My favorite wine is whatever has a pretty label at Costco.) I didn't get fall-down drunk, mind you, although that might not have been a bad idea under the circumstances. My two glasses of wine were just enough wine to magnify the sadness, which obviously wasn't the original plan.

The next few weeks certainly didn't play out the way we expected with our brilliant FLNC plan. First there was the birthday contact (initiated by me) and next there was the *I need to visit Caly* contact (initiated by Tristan). Since the NC part of FLNC had obviously gone to hell after only a few weeks, Tristan thought that it would be okay to come and see the pup. Full disclosure: she sent me a text message (I cannot emphasize enough how this technology is clearly one of the wonders of my world) asking if I was home. I said that no, I wasn't home but I'd be home in an hour. She explained that she was close to the house, would be dropping by to see Caly, and would be gone before I got home. By now it had been a month since I'd seen her; I needed to see her. What followed next was a tiny bit deceptive, but not a big deal in my book. I got in my car and went home to see my child. Our little reunion was a little odd, maybe a bit strained, but it was okay. We sat on the floor and made small talk while Caly licked Tristan in the ear (I know that's gross, but that's what Caly does—she's a dog). And then Tristan left.

My next contact with Tristan was about money and school; our money, her school. As always, it was via text. She wanted to know if the money/allowance situation would change if she did an about-face and decided to pursue a bachelor's degree instead of a paramedic certification. She had found out that Starbucks offered a pretty substantial subsidy for their employees seeking a bachelor's degree, and she thought it wise to put the paramedic track on hold and pursue the bachelor's for the next few years. Her interests were in political science and history, two perfect fits for her. She took a stab and asked for the next sixteen-months' allowance up front, which we declined. She'd need to get it in smaller chunks as agreed with the FLNC. All she could do was ask, right?

After that my next contact was when I learned through the grapevine (i.e., Grandma) that Tristan had an emergency, but no worries because it was handled. How do you throw a control freak mama into a tizzy? Tell her that her child had an emergency, but it's all okay now so no need to worry. I contacted Tristan, certain that we had a bona fide emergency on our hands. Turns out, the emergency was a dead car battery. Small potatoes, as Curt's dad would say.

It was pretty much hit-or-miss by then. Tristan would text me to see if Caly was at home (where else would she be, she's a dog), I'd text her to tell her she had mail at the house, and so on. On

Halloween I sent Tristan some photos of Caly looking particularly adorable in her costume, and the next thing I knew it was two weeks before Thanksgiving. I reached out to see if she'd be joining us for dinner, but she was working that day, so she declined. I'm sure she volunteered to work; family holidays can be difficult to say the least during FLNC.

Actually, the last two sentences are the condensed version of the Thanksgiving dinner that wasn't. When I texted Tristan to ask if she would join us for dinner, the response I got was quite unexpected. She let me know that she would not be joining us for Thanksgiving or any other family gathering until Curt and I apologized. Apologize? For what? Tristan insisted that we apologize for sending her an email that she was "dead to us." Her words, I kid you not. I pulled up the aforementioned email, re-read it eighty-seven times, and could find nothing to indicate that Tristan was dead to us or anyone else. Yes, we had invoked the FLNC, but for God's sake it was the only way any of us were going to survive this relationship that we hoped to salvage some day.

Game on. I had to go deeper with this one. This is exactly, word for word, what I sent to her (via text, of course): "You were invited to join the family. No one is 'dead' to anyone. I will not tolerate tension or controversy on Thanksgiving. Anyone who can be polite and pleasant is always welcome. You are not owed an apology. Your dad and I made a choice based on our unwillingness to accept the anger that you direct toward us when we are together. If you can join us without that anger, then we would love to see you. If not, then we understand your choice." She sent me a screen shot of the "dead to us" email. I read it AGAIN, forwards then backwards, and there is no mention of us killing her off.

So, I sent this: "You came to see Caly and were pleasant. Based on that I had hoped that we might be able to spend Thanksgiving together with equal pleasantness. Understand that we are in no way indicating we will tolerate unpleasant behavior. Invitation extended. The choice is yours. No other discussion is necessary." For good or for bad, she took me at my word, and there was no other discussion. Crickets. Until Thanksgiving morning, when I couldn't take it anymore. The vision of her eating a frozen turkey dinner was too much, I had to try one more time. So, Thanksgiving morning I sent one final turkey-day text: "Hope you'll decide to join us." Again, crickets.

SO MUCH LOSS

Wouldn't it be wonderful if childhood was the stuff of movies? I mean real family movies like *The Sound of Music* and *Mary Poppins*, not *Meet the Fockers* and *National Lampoon's Christmas Vacation* (both of which are incredibly funny, but let's face it—not exactly the picture-perfect family you'd long to trade places with). Childhood should be filled with laughter and love, unicorns and rainbows. Children should not have to deal with death, they shouldn't have to grieve. But life isn't the movies, is it? In real life we can't always shield children from the loss of those they love and the grief that follows.

Anna, like so many others, experienced death when she was a child. She lost an uncle and a grandmother, and she lost a few great-grandparents. That was hard, as it's always hard when you lose someone in your family. But, at the same time, it's the circle of life, isn't it? The older generation passes, and the younger generation is left. That's the way it's supposed to be.

We all know that the time will come when we'll need to say goodbye to grandparents and parents, and then the time will come when our own children will have to say goodbye to us. That's how it's supposed to work. But things don't always work the way they're supposed to, and circles sometimes lose their shape. By the time Tristan (she was still Anna then) was twelve years old she had experienced more loss than any child should have; her circle had been absolutely mangled.

Remember earlier when I mentioned how Tristan as a little girl used to tell us that she was going to marry Chris' best friend? That young man's name was Bobby, and he was one of a kind. Bobby was an only child (I could so relate to him), and Chris loved hanging around Bobby's house because it was calm. The two of them could do what they wanted without sibling interruptus. Bobby seemed to love hanging around our house because it was anything but calm. We always want what we don't have, right? He fit in perfectly with all of the noise and confusion that you find in a big family. I'm sure he was happy when it was time to leave our asylum and go home, but when he was with us he fit right in like one of the family.

It was actually fourteen-year-old Bobby who came up with the idea that he and Tristan, who was a four-year-old Anna at the time, would get married when she came of age. At first she resisted, but Bobby was irresistible so eventually she gave in. He'd walk through the door of our house and loudly announce some version of, "Anna, I'm here! It's me, Bobby, your boyfriend. Remember, we're gonna get married." Who could resist that? That lasted for a few years, until she was old enough to be embarrassed by the whole thing.

When Anna was ten years old, Bobby was in a tragic accident. He spent two weeks in the ICU before he passed away. I went every day, but I never took her. The ICU had a very strict *no visitors under age fourteen allowed* rule, and I'm an obsessive rule follower. And so I never took her. I screwed up. If only I'd have broken the rule; I should have taken her to say goodbye. She's reminded me of it more times than I can count, and I've apologized just as many times. But not taking her will forever be one of the top things on my list of things I would change if only I could go back and change them.

We're supposed to learn from our mistakes, aren't we? But

tragedy often throws us into reaction mode; we lose our sense of logic, and we forget the lessons we've learned. I should have learned from Bobby, but I didn't. Two years after Bobby passed away Tristan had to face another tragic loss. This time it was Andrew's dear friend, Will. He came into our lives when he was fourteen; Andrew was sixteen, and Tristan was a ten-year-old Anna. It's somewhat ironic that she lost Bobby when she was ten, but she got Will the same year.

Will was a two-year fixture in our house. He was with us for dinner (OMG he could eat like no other teenage boy I've ever seen), for long weekends away, and even for family vacations. There was no marriage plan for the two of them, but Anna loved having Will around. Early one morning the phone rang; Will's mom was calling to ask me to bring Andrew to the hospital ASAP. Will was in intensive care and the doctors weren't sure he'd make it. It was prom weekend. Andrew had just seen Will, only about twelve hours before.

Will passed away after less than two days in the hospital. And, again, I screwed up. When the phone call came, the call that said *get here quickly, something horrible has happened and he may not make it,* I sent Tristan to school and took Andrew to the hospital. She knew that something was wrong with Will, but she didn't know how awful it was. I didn't know how awful it was until I got there. He was gone in less than forty-eight hours. It was so quick. And I didn't take her to the hospital. Of course, there was still the *fourteen years or older* rule, but this time that's not what kept me from taking her. I couldn't bear the thought of her seeing that big goofball hooked up to tubes and machines, so I didn't take her. She was twelve.

This was twice in two years; it was too much. And I majorly screwed up. Another thing added to the list of things I'd give anything to change, another thing added to the list of colossal parental screw ups. Another thing that I can never make right, no matter how many times I apologize. Another thing that Tristan will likely never forgive me for. Who can blame her?

CHAPTER 22

THE REARVIEW

Our culture has accepted two huge lies. The first is that if you disagree with someone's lifestyle, you must fear or hate them. The second is that to love someone means you agree with everything they believe or do. Both are nonsense. You don't have to compromise convictions to be compassionate.

~ Rick Warren

People fascinate me; words fascinate me. People and the words they choose fascinate me the most. I'm usually careful with my words (notice I said usually). I like to think before I speak, as I know from personal experience how easy it is to say something that you'll always regret but that you can never take back. When I think back at some of the idiotic things that have come out of my mouth, I just hope that I'm the only one who remembers.

When Tristan was eighteen, in the midst of the angst and turmoil that had become our lives, she said something to me that I'll never forget. Something I hope and pray she never believed to be true for a single moment. Here's what she said: I never wanted her, she was a mistake, and why didn't I get an abortion when I found out I was pregnant. I was dumbfounded. Never, in the history of wanted children, did I think there had been a more wanted child. Sure, she was God's little surprise, but she was God's tremendous gift. She was never a mistake, she was always wanted, and she has always been loved.

Tristan's lifestyle as a transgender male I can accept. Admittedly, though, I may never understand it. There were no signs. Why weren't there signs? That's my question: why no signs? She was a girly girl. She wanted to wear princess dresses and makeup. She played with dolls and stuffed animals, not trucks and tools. Her favorite thing to do when she was about seven years old was to dress up as a rockstar and pretend to be Sodapop, her alter ego. Mallory and her friend, Georgia would spend hours helping Sodapop come to life with elaborate hair, makeup, and costumes. Sodapop was clearly a chick rocker. Am I stereotyping? If I am, then how can I not?

I grew up in a time when there were two genders, male and female. There were males who were feminine and females who were masculine. There were no lists of gender-related definitions to help us understand someone's gender identity. Now we have lists of terms to help us understand gender identity, and we sure do need them. Because you never know when one day your not-so-little-anymore girl will tell you—totally out of the blue—that she's never really been your little girl at all. And she'll likely expect you to just go with it. And you'll try to process it, but it's all happening so fast. And you'll use the wrong name and the wrong pronouns. And you will mourn, and you will grieve, and you will cry. And it's likely that you will not understand. But, still, you'll love your not-so-little girl just as much as you loved her when she was your little girl. But, she's not your girl anymore, is she? That's what she tells you and thank goodness you have lists and social media groups and Google to help you survive as you try your best to understand how life changed in the blink of an eye.

I wish I could share half of the information that Google has bestowed upon me in my quest for transgender understanding, but I'll narrow it down to the one article that fascinates me most, probably because I relate to it so completely. The article is titled, *Why Is Transgender Identity on the Rise Among Teens? A new study of social contagion raises important clinical and ethical questions.* It was written by a professor at McGill University, Samuel Veissière, Ph.D. According to his bio, Dr. Veissière is an "anthropologist and cognitive scientist who studies the interaction between cognition, culture, and cooperative human behavior." The first time I read the article I could almost hear Roberta Flack singing . . . *telling my whole life with his words, killing me softly with his song.* Dr. V. may not have written the article about me, but he sure was telling my life with his words:

> "In a recent survey of 250 families whose children developed symptoms of gender dysphoria during or right
> after puberty, Debra Littman, a physician and professor of behavioral science at Brown University, found that over 80 percent of the youth in her sample were female at birth. Littman's study reported many other surprising findings. To meet the diagnostic criteria for gender dysphoria, a child typically needs to have shown observable characteristics of the condition prior to puberty, such as 'a strong rejection of typically feminine or masculine toys,' or 'a strong resistance to wearing typically feminine or masculine clothes.' Again, eighty percent of the parents in the study reported observing none of these early signs in their children."

The plot thickens again: First, many of the youth in the survey had been directly exposed to one or more peers who had recently "come out" as trans. Next, 63.5 percent of the parents reported that in the time just before announcing they were trans, their child had exhibited a marked increase in Internet and social media consumption. Following popular YouTubers who discussed their transition thus emerged as a common factor in many of the cases. After the youth came out, an increase in distress, conflict with parents, and voiced antagonism toward heterosexual people and non-transgender people (known as "cis" or "cisgender") was also frequently reported. This animosity was also described as extending to "males, white people, gay and lesbian (non-transgender) people." The view adopted by trans youth, as summed up by one parent, seemed to be that:

> "In general, cis-gendered people are considered evil and unsupportive, regardless of their actual views on the topic. To be heterosexual, comfortable with the gender you were assigned at birth, and non-minority places you in the 'most evil' of categories with this group of friends. Statement of opinions by the evil cis-gendered population are consider phobic and discriminatory and are generally discounted as unenlightened.

Littman raises cautions about encouraging young people's desire to transition in all instances. From the cases reviewed in her study, she concluded that what she terms *rapid-onset gender dysphoria*' (ROGD) appears to be a novel condition that emerges from cohort and contagion effects and novel social pressures. From this perspective, ROGD likely exhibits an aetiology and epidemiology that is distinct from the 'classical' cases of gender dysphoria documented in the DSM (Diagnostic and Statistical Manual of Mental Disorders).

Littman hypothesizes that ROGD can be cast as a *maladaptive coping mechanism* for other underlying mental health issues such as trauma or social maladjustment, but also for other exceptional traits like high IQ and giftedness. The peer support, prestige, and identity leveraged by the youth who proudly come out as trans certainly appears to be protective in their circles. As Littman's study shows, this social signaling strategy also comes with strong disadvantages, particularly as it increases conflict between trans youth and the 'cis' majority of the population, which, tellingly, includes a majority of the LGBT community."

Finally! I'm not the only one who questions ROGD. Maybe I'm not crazy to question Tristan's sudden transgender identity. There are others like me out there, somewhere, who struggle as I do. We question the influence of social media, of peers, of life trauma on these super-intelligent young people who wake up one day and tell us that they are no longer the gender that they were born with.

But, at the end of the day, guess what that article and so many others like it really mean? Nothing. They mean absolutely nothing. Reading an article like that offers the most temporary kind of euphoria to a parent searching for answers. I read it and was elated —for ten seconds and then I realized that it changes nothing. As comforting as it is to know I'm not alone in my confusion, it doesn't really change a thing, does it? I had Anna for almost two decades, and I don't think she's coming back.

I admit it, I'm selfish when it comes to this whole thing. I love Tristan, and I still want Anna back. And what would I say if she walked through the door and said, "Guess what, mom? I've decided to be Anna again. Tristan really isn't working for me anymore." I'd say, "Welcome back." But for now, who knows what lies ahead? Madame Sophia is long gone, and I realized years ago that if you're looking for a crystal ball you might as well settle for a Magic 8 Ball because the answers will be just as telling: *Cannot Predict Now, It Is Uncertain, Reply Hazy Try Again.*

The Magic 8 Ball is actually right, isn't it? The future is unpredictable, uncertain, and hazy. Twenty years ago, I prayed to know who was supposed to fill the empty seat at the kitchen table, and nineteen years ago Anna filled it. But it's empty again. It's Tristan's seat now, not Anna's, and Tristan left it empty the third Thanksgiving *after*. That empty seat was almost too much. Almost, but almost doesn't count. And so, again, I pray.

But I don't pray for someone to fill the empty seat; it belongs to Tristan. I pray that she'll be happy, that she'll love herself, and that life's cruelties will pass her by. I pray that her friends will be close and her enemies will be distant—and that she'll know which is which. I pray that she'll take her seat at the table.

NO ONE'S PERFECT

When I decided to write this, I told almost no one. Curt knew, a few girlfriends (beans spilled over a glass of wine), and no one else. Invariably, each girlfriend said the same exact thing the moment they found out what I was writing. *Will you use your real name? You won't, will you? I mean, you can't use your real name.* My answer was always the same: *Yes, I'll use my real name. How can I write a book that promises no BS and then not use my real name?* Every one of them accepted my answer and moved on except one.

My friend, Peg, totally called me out on it. She basically said that no, I couldn't use my real name and to do so would be a colossal mistake. Pray, tell? I was intrigued, and she explained. She pointed out that, for the twenty-plus years that we'd been friends, my purpose in life seemed (in her opinion) to be to project perfection. WHAT? I was not one of those perfect people with perfect families that you see on social media. No friggin' way.

But, the more she talked, the more I wondered. She sugarcoated nothing, and she had examples to back up her theory (which I will not share here, just in case she's right and perhaps I really do want everyone to think I'm perfect). Her point was this: I had never in my entire life opened myself up and exposed my struggles or my heartaches or my challenges. I came across as someone who had everything under control. I had wanted everyone in my circle to think that life in my world was picture-perfect. I was shocked. And, since we were having a leisurely girls-night-out dinner and were in no rush, I had plenty of time to hear more. She talked, I listened. She described me as others saw me, and not at all as I saw myself. Of course, she was kind as she pointed out my imperfect quest for the appearance of perfection. And she certainly left me with much to think about, not the least of which was whether using my real name as I share my struggles with the world was the right decision. But I promised no BS, didn't I?

EPILOGUE

THE HOPE

The trouble is, you think you have time.

~ Jack Kornfield, *Buddha's Little Instruction Book*

———————

Tristan offered something of a compromise at Christmas. This was our third Christmas *after* and our first Christmas with FLNC (firm love no contact, just in case you need a reminder). The compromise was this: Tristan would come to Grandma and Grandpa's house for Christmas Eve dinner (my parents, as was our family tradition), and would work at Starbucks on Christmas Day. This would be the first time she'd seen Curt in four months; he was the only one who'd come even close to achieving FLNC. I took her gifts to Grandma and Grandpa's house and let her know that it was okay to open them there or take them back to her apartment. There were quite a few gifts; in my mind there was no way that FLNC meant no gifts at Christmas.

So, what do you give your AFAB transgender child for Christmas when you're in the midst of FLNC? It actually wasn't that hard. She had mentioned months ago that she needed a vacuum, and I knew that was a safe gift since there was no way she'd have gotten one yet. What teenager buys themselves a vacuum? There were the impractical things, the things I knew she'd like but certainly didn't need (a leather journal, a fancy pen, some craft kit things—craft stuff can be gender neutral, and Tristan still loved her craft stuff).

The rest of the Christmas gifts were something of an olive branch on my part. There was the quite masculine leather keychain stamped with her new initials. And there were clothes—men's clothes. Sweaters, pants, socks, all from the men's department. She opened them on Christmas Eve, then went on her way to prepare for a holly jolly Christmas Day slinging coffee. Yes, there are people who cannot do without their Starbucks, even on Christmas Day.

A few days later Tristan offered her own olive branch in the way of a text message (shocker) to thank me for the Christmas gifts. To quote her, I "nailed it." It seemed like we were taking baby steps, so maybe now we'd moved to FLMC (firm love minimal contact). Whatever it was, I was willing to take it. Getting random texts here and there was better than wondering day after day if your child was lying in a ditch (why do mamas always envision their children lying in a ditch just because they haven't talked to them in twenty-four hours?).

Since the FLMC thing seemed to work for us at Christmas I asked Tristan if she'd be interested in coming over on New Year's Eve to take Caly out for a potty break since Curt and I wanted to go out and ring in the new year. After all, Tristan had once been a professional pet sitter. In true Tristan fashion she negotiated a holiday pay rate as well as a pizza to seal the deal. I would have expected nothing less from the master of negotiation. We invited her for a New Year's Day lunch, probably pushing it a little, but she had to work anyway so the answer was no—Starbucks is serious business, 24/7/365 lest you've forgotten.

We hear from her every few days, and I think this FLMC thing is working for all of us, at least for now. Sometimes she'll come over for dinner, and sometimes she just wants to tell us that she thinks we need a second pup to keep Caly company. Sometimes she wants her membership number to American Airlines because she's off to right the wrongs of the world at another rally in a distant state.

And I have hope, because remember, I'm ever the optimist. I hope that soon Tristan and I will figure this thing out together. I hope that it gets easier, for both of us. I hope, as the Magic 8 Ball says, *You May Rely On It.*

AFTERWORD

When I decided to write about my journey as the mom of a trans-gender teenager, I kept it to myself (and Curt) for a long time. Writing was my therapy, and it brought out the emotions that you'd expect from good therapy. Then came the questions, because good therapy should lead to questions. One of the questions was this: what do I do with this stuff that I'm writing? That's the questions that turned the "stuff" into a book. As I started to get brave and share my writing adventure with a (very) few close friends, the feedback was this—there are other parents who are walking in my shoes who might benefit from my words. So I wrote a book.

The book was completed in seven months, but it took another two months for me to get the courage to tell Tristan (the child formerly known as Anna) about the book. At one point during that two month gap I asked myself another question: should I try and publish? It would have been so much easier to save the file and keep it to myself. But, easy wasn't an option. I told Tristan about the book, braced myself for whatever reaction came my way, and offered to share an electronic copy. And the reaction? The short version is that the book has the Tristan Blaine seal of approval. When I offered to share it I was clear about two things, so Tristan knew what to expect: 1) there are parts of the book where Tristan looks like a brat, and 2) there are parts of the book where I look like an asshole.

The Tristan seal of approval was key; without it the book would never have gone to print.

GLOSSARY OF TERMS

- **AFAB** - Assigned Female at Birth.
- **AMAB** - Assigned Male at Birth.
- **Agender** - Does not identify with any gender.
- **Androgynous** - Has both feminine and masculine traits.
- **Asexual ("ace")** - Has no sexual attraction to others.
- **Binding** - Wrapping breasts (AFAB) with tight compression garment to hide the breasts.
- **Bisexual** - Someone who is attracted to both masculine and/or feminine individuals.
- **Cisgender** - Someone whose gender identity matches their birth gender. The opposite of transgender.
- **Deadname** - The name given at birth of someone who then changes their name.
- **FTM** - Female to Male. Referred to as a transgender male. Born a female, identifies as a male.
- **FTX** - Female to X. A transgender person (AFAB) who is gender expansive but does not identify as transgender male.
- **Gay** - A person who is attracted to people of the same gender.

- **GAS** - Gender Affirming Surgery. A surgical procedure that helps align a person's body with their gender identity.
- **Gender Dysphoria** - The mental distress felt by a person whose body does not match their gender identity.
- **Gender Expansive** - The feeling of existing psychologically between genders. Some gender-expansive individuals identify as a man or a woman, some identify as neither, and others identify as a mix of both.
- **Gender Expression** - How someone presents their gender (with clothes, hairstyle, etc).
- **Gender Identity** - The gender with which a person identifies.
- **Intersex** - Someone whose sex chromosomes are not typically male or female. Born with genitalia that is neither typically male or female.
- **LGBTQIA+** - Lesbian, Gay, Bisexual, Transgender, Queer or Questioning, Intersex, Asexual, and more.
- **Misgender** - When someone is referred to by the wrong gender.
- **MTF** - Male to Female. Referred to as a transgender female. Born a male, identifies as a female.
- **MTX** - Male to X. A transgender person (AMAB) who is gender expansive but does not identify as female.
- **Non-Binary** - A transgender person who does not identify strictly as male or as female. They may identify as agender, genderqueer, non-binary, or as another gender all together.
- **Pansexual** - Someone who is sexually attracted to those of any gender (regardless of sex, gender, identity, and orientation).
- **Passing** - A transgender person being perceived (by others) as the gender in which they identify.

- **Pronouns** - He/him/his, she/her/hers, they/them/theirs, ze/zim/zirs, and more.
- **ROGD** - Rapid onset gender dysphoria.
- **Stealth** - A transgender person who is living their life as the gender they identify as. They do not disclose their birth gender to other people, publicly or privately.
- **Transgender** - Someone who identifies as a gender other than their birth gender. Includes gender expansive persons that identify as neither male nor female. Not every transgender person chooses to physically present their body as their identified gender (ex: AFAB may choose NOT to present themselves bodily as male).
- **Transition** - Someone who is socially, legally, and/or medically changing their gender expression to coincide with their gender identity.
- **Transsexual** - Someone who is medically changing or has changed their body to match their gender identity.

REFERENCES

Foreword

Ray Donovan. Showtime, 2013-2020.

Chapter 1

Holy Bible: Contemporary English Version (American Bible Society, 1995), Isaiah 44:2a.

Chapter 2

Mark Hoppus (Blink 182), Quotefancy, https://quotefancy.com/quote/1243859/Mark-Hoppus-Everything-in-high-school-seems-like-the-most-important-thing-that-s-ever.

All My Children. ABC, 1970-2011.

DINKLES® is a *trademark* of Up-Front Footwear, Inc..

CHICK-FIL-A® is a registered *trademark* and service mark of *CFA PROPERTIES, INC. ("CFA Properties")*.

STARBUCKS COFFEE is a *trademark* of *STARBUCKS* CORPORATION.

DCI is a *trademark* of *DRUM CORPS INTERNATIONAL*, INC.

JCPENNEY is a *trademark* of J. C. Penney Corporation, Inc.

COSTCO WHOLESALE is a *trademark* of *Costco* Wholesale Membership, Inc.

REI is a *trademark* of Recreational Equipment, Inc.

AMAZON is a *trademark* of *Amazon*.com, Inc.

Chapter 3

Graham Brown, Goodreads, Quotes>Quotable Quote, https://www.goodreads.com/quotes/6965228-life-is-about-choices-some-we-regret-some-we-re-proud.

The Oxygen Channel is a *trademark* of *NBC UNIVERSAL MEDIA*, LLC.

HOLIDAY INN is a *trademark* of *HOLIDAY INNS*, INC.

TYLENOL is a *trademark* of JOHNSON & JOHNSON.

BAND-AID is a *trademark* of JOHNSON & JOHNSON.

NETFLIX is a *trademark* of *Netflix*, Inc.

Chapter 4

Lewis Carroll, *Alice in Wonderland*. Goodreads, https://www.goodreads.com/quotes/131294-it-s-no-use-going-back-to-yesterday-because-i-was

Chapter 5

Wes Angelozzi, Quote Catalog, https://quotecatalog.com/quote/wes-angelozzi-go-and-love-som-EpREGm7/

GIRL SCOUTS is a trademark of *Girl Scouts OF THE United States OF AMERICA*

GOOGLE is a trademark of *GOOGLE INC.*

Cecilia A. Essau, Delyse Hutchinson, *Adolescent Addiction, 2008,* "Alcohol Use, Abuse, and Dependence," Science Direct, 2008, https://www.sciencedirect.com/science/article/pii/B978012373625350005X which cites *Barnes*, Reifman, Farrell, & Dintcheff, 2000, "Parental and peer influences on the onset of heavier drinking among adolescents," U.S. National Library of Medicine National Institutes of Health, 2000, https://www.ncbi.nlm.nih.gov/pubmed/9598712

Tamara Hill, "10 Signs Of Having An Emotionally Unstable/Unavailable Parent," last modified March 6, 2018, https://blogs.psychcentral.com/caregivers/2018/01/10-signs-of-having-an-emotionally-unstable-unavailable-parent/

Yulande Roxburgh, "How to Be Emotionally Available to Your Kids," last modified November 8, 2017, https://cleverlittlemonkey.co.za/emotionally-available-to-your-kids/

Chapter 6

Fred Rogers, Goodreads, Quotes>Quotable Quote, https://www.goodreads.com/quotes/180952-love-isn-t-a-state-of-perfect-caring-it-is-an

Chapter 7

Mark Twain, Goodreads, Quotes>Quotable Quote, https://www.goodreads.com/quotes/545616-to-a-man-with-a-hammer-everything-looks-like-a

Wikipedia; Wikipedia's "Detransition" entry; Wikipedia's entry on the term *Detransition*

Wikipedia; Wikipedia's "Desistance" entry; Wikipedia's entry on the term *Desistance*

Chapter 8

Nora Ephron, "I Feel Bad About My Neck: And Other Thoughts on Being a Woman." Goodreads, Quotes>Quotable Quote, https://www.goodreads.com/quotes/175728-when-your-children-are-teenagers-it-s-important-to-have-a

BAND-AID is a *trademark* of JOHNSON & JOHNSON.

Chapter 9

Joyce Carole Oates, "After the Wreck, I Picked Myself Up, Spread My Wings, and Flew Away," Goodreads, Quotes>Quotable Quote, https://www.goodreads.com/quotes/52161-see-people-come-into-your-life-for-a-reason-they

My Big Fat Greek Wedding. Motion picture. Directed by Joel Zwick. New York City, NY: IFC Films, 2002.

Number One Fan

DISNEY is a *trademark* of *DISNEY* ENTERPRISES, INC.

Lion King. Motion picture. Directed by Roger Allers and Rob Minkoff. Burbank, CA: Walt Disney Pictures/Buena Vista Pictures, 1994.

The Phantom of the Opera. Motion picture. Directed by Joel Schumacher. Burbank, CA: Warner Brothers Pictures, 2004.

Emmy Possum, Patrick Wilson. 2004. "Think of Me." Track 2 on *The Phantom of the Opera Soundtrack.* Sony Masterworks, compact disc.

Chapter 11

Kevin Heath, https://www.passiton.com/inspirational-quotes/4692-wherever-there-is-a-human-in-need-there-is-an

Chapter 12

Victor Hugo, "Les Miserables" Goodreads, Quotes>Quotable Quote, https://www.goodreads.com/quotes/10095-even-the-darkest-night-will-end-and-the-sun-will

Kendra Cherry, "Differences Between Psychologists and Psychiatrists," last modified December 12, 2019, https://www.verywellmind.com/psychologists-vs-psychiatrists-what-is-the-difference-2795761

The Odd Couple. Television series. CBS, 1970-1975.

Chapter 13

Wikipedia; Wikipedia's "Serenity Prayer" entry; Wikipedia's entry on the term *Serenity Prayer* by Reinhold Niebuhr.

The Mayo Clinic, "Masculinizing Hormone Therapy ," last modified April 14, 2020, https://www.mayoclinic.org/tests-procedures/ftm-hormone-therapy/about/pac-20385099

Chapter 14

The Police. 1983. "Wrapped Around Your Finger." Track 9 on *Synchronicity*. A&M Records, compact disc.

Chapter 15

Robert Frost, Goodreads, Quotes>Quotable Quote, https://www.goodreads.com/quotes/258-in-three-words-i-can-sum-up-everything-i-ve-learned

Chapter 16

Lucius Annaeus Seneca, Goodreads, Quotes>Quotable Quote, https://www.goodreads.com/quotes/490670-every-new-beginning-comes-from-some-other-beginning-s-end

Christmas Stockings

SNICKERS is a *trademark* of MARS, INCORPORATED.

Chapter 17

Amira Ahmed, *I Have Stories to Tell*, Xlibris US (December 27, 2019)

Chapter 18

Jaimie Anderson, Goodreads, Quotes>Quotable Quote, https://www.goodreads.com/author/quotes/3395454.Jamie_Anderson

Mere Abrams, "Top Surgery," November 7, 2017, https://www.healthline.com/health/transgender/top-surgery

Benjie Jones, "The staggering costs of being transgender in the US, where even patients with health insurance can face six-figure bills," July 10, 2019, https://www.businessinsider.com/transgender-medical-care-surgery-expensive-2019-6

Chapter 19

Martin Luther King Jr., Goodreads, Quotes>Quotable Quote, https://www.goodreads.com/quotes/37292-we-must-accept-finite-disappointment-but-never-lose-infinite-hope

Chapter 20

Kid Cudi. 2009. "Soundtrack 2 My Life." Track 2 on *Soundtrack 2 My Life*. Dream On/GOOD/Universal Motown, studio album.

Chapter 21

Keanu Reeves, Goodreads, Quotes>Quotable Quote, https://www.goodreads.com/quotes/7137953-grief-changes-shape-but-it-never-ends

So Much Loss

Sound of Music. Motion Picture. Directed by Robert Wise. Los Angeles, CA: 20th Century Fox, 1965.

Mary Poppins. Motion Picture. Directed by Robert Stevenson. Los Angeles, CA: Walt Disney/Buena Vista Distributions, 1964.

Meet the Fockers. Motion Picture. Directed by Jay Roach. Universal City, CA: Universal Pictures (North America) DreamWorks Pictures (International), 2004.

National Lampoon's Christmas Vacation. Motion Picture. Directed by Jeremiah S. Chechik. Burbank, CA: Warner Brothers, 1989.

Chapter 22

Rick Warren, Goodreads, Quotes>Quotable Quote, https://www.goodreads.com/quotes/601712-our-culture-has-accepted-two-huge-lies-the-first-is

Samuel Paul Veissière, Ph.D., "Why Is Transgender Identity on the Rise Among Teens?" November 28, 2018, https://www.psychologytoday.com/us/blog/culture-mind-and-brain/201811/why-is-transgender-identity-the-rise-among-teens

Roberta Flack. 1972. "Killing Me Softly," Track 1 on *Killing Me Softly*. Atlantic Records, vinyl record.

MAGIC 8 BALL is a *trademark* of MATTEL, INC.

Epilogue

Jack Kornfield, "Buddha's Little Instruction Book," Goodreads, Quotes>Quotable Quote, https://www.goodreads.com/quotes/669971-the-trouble-is-you-think-you-have-time

AMERICAN AIRLINES is a *trademark* of *American Airlines*, Inc.

ABOUT THE AUTHOR

Patti Hornstra is a native of Richmond, Virginia, and a graduate of Virginia Commonwealth University with degrees in Marketing and Business Education. Her days are filled with adventure as a real estate broker, while her nights are spent fixated on becoming a writer. This is her first book. She married the love of her life, Curtis, in 1987 and together they have raised four children. They have adjusted nicely to life as empty nesters and eagerly await life's next great adventure. Patti enjoys VCU Basketball (GO RAMS!), traveling to new places, and spending time at the "Rivah."

CPSIA information can be obtained
at www.ICGtesting.com
Printed in the USA
FSHW020817201020
74887FS